Artisan Perfumery
or
Being Led by the Nose

Alec Lawless

First Published in 2009 by
Boronia Souk Ltd.
Unit 16, Griffin Mill,
London Road,
Thrupp,
Stroud,
Glos GL5 2AZ.
info@essentially-me.co.uk

Layout by Shaun Hodge
Printed by Remous Limited, Milborne Port, Dorset DT9 5EP
www.remous.com

ISBN 978-0-9562137-0-9

Cover picture: Detail from centre of painting. Flowers like jasmine, lilies and tuberose are dependent on the moth for pollination and communicate with it by exuding a sweet heavy scent that mimics the pheromones of the moth. Some moths can smell a single bloom from six miles downwind. The reason these blooms are white is so they are able to reflect light from the moon and the stars to further aid the moth to find and pollinate them. These white, heady, sweet, floral aromas provide some of the most exotic, ethereal and romantic scents.

In Memory of B. D.
The Greatest Nose of Them All

Illustrations

Contents

Introduction

The two questions that I am most frequently asked in relation to making perfume are, "How did you get into that?" and "What's the most expensive oil?" Predilection and life circumstances are the answer to the first question. I probably inherited a keen sense of smell from my mother, who knew whether I had been smoking as a child as soon as I walked into the house, even if she was in another room. I was introduced to essential oils when I met Julia and, shortly after that, Aqua Oleum and a daughter emerged from our union. Julia established herself as a successful author, writing quality books about essential oils and I developed our company.

We had left London and moved to the country and shortly after that I quit my job and spent two very scary years trying to make enough money to pay the bills. Thankfully, the company got on its feet and provided us with a decent living. Familiarity with the oils would have been impossible to avoid as my working life was spent surrounded by them. Initially, the business was in our small end of terrace cottage so there was no escaping the smells, even at night. I learnt a lot from my trading relationships with suppliers, even though some of them proved to be unreliable and dishonest.

Having spent three years in the Merchant Navy, I had travelled extensively and seen many countries before globalisation had really developed its neutralising effect on diverse cultures. As the oils I was buying literally came from all over the world, I did have a sense of connection with many distant shores. Being agricultural products, many of the oils had a long tradition of cultivation and extraction which added another layer of interest. Both factors were heightened by the stories I heard from suppliers and producers about circumstances at origin. These could involve eccentric families, tribal disputes, wars, smuggling, swindling, folklore, extreme climatic conditions and changes in legislation. All these factors can and do affect quality, reliability of the supply chain and price, creating quite a colourful, entertaining and sometimes frustrating trading environment.

Two other major factors which 'got me into it' are food and wine. I started cooking when I was fourteen. We were on a family camping holiday in Devon and my father used to take us fishing in a small wooden boat. One day we took an Asian family who were staying on the same campsite with us. The women stayed behind and when we returned with our catch for a fish supper we were greeted by chicken curry. I was proud of my dad because in 1973 not everyone was so welcoming to Asian families. My mother had helped in the preparation and after that holiday curry night became a weekly occurrence. Making curry seemed an incredibly cool thing to do and it was the hook that got me into cooking. I regularly spend three hours a day in the kitchen.

I make no apology for my frequent digressions into the world of wine, as it is so interconnected with the world of fine fragrance. For commercial reasons it is almost impossible to get trained as a perfumer. However, professional wine courses are accessible to the public and are an excellent systematic olfactory training which can help wake up and refine the nose. Certain red wines remain the most aromatically complex experiences in my life.

The final ingredient in making fragrances is passion. As Louis Armstrong said when asked what rhythm is, "Maam, if you don't know, you ain't got it."

In answer to the second question, the most expensive is oil is extracted from infected agarwood, which is also known as aloewood. It is a flowering evergreen tree (Aquilaria agallocha) from Southeast Asia whose scent derives from an aromatic resin produced by the tree as an immune response to a fungal infection. The fungus is so rare that the infection only arises rarely which, combined with the low yield of the oil and demand for the wood, accounts for the price. The wood itself is used for costly incense. I have heard stories of agarwood farms being surrounded with barbed wire and armed guards to deter poachers. I bought a small piece of the infected wood from an incense maker in China. It is not very heavily infected but I am convinced it is genuine. If I remove a splinter and warm it over a flame, it releases a beautifully complex, sweet and heady aroma reminiscent of sandalwood with hints of rose, precious resins, leather and an Arabian bazaar. This piece of wood was part of my inspiration for creating a perfume called Souk. The Hindi word for incense is agarbath because agarwood has been traditionally prized for centuries. The oil was also contained in a legendary Arabian fragrance called Owd, Oud or Awd. I have been offered oil on several occasions in India that the purveyors called agarwood at a price equivalent to £150,000 per kg (November 2008). I have yet to come across oil that I believe is genuinely distilled from infected agarwood.

I begin this book with an historical overview of aromatic raw materials and perfume. I am not attempting a definitive history because this has been covered much more comprehensively elsewhere. I am more interested in a brief summary for the sake of completion and putting the contemporary fragrance situation into historical context. The first part of this chapter was used to inform artist Fiona Owen in order to help her produce her narrative masterpiece, which I commissioned. It is illustrated later in this book. The second chapter covers some of the issues around sourcing genuine natural raw materials and is largely a response to repeated questions from customers over a twenty one year period. For chapter three I thought it made sense to write in detail about a single oil in order to try and convey some of the richness alluded to already.

Chapter four contains reflections around the natural synthetic debate, which in some quarters is as emotive as debates around foxhunting can get. Some natural perfumers across the pond insist that in order to call a perfume 'natural' it should be based in grain alcohol which is preferably organic. In the UK we do not enjoy access to perfume alcohol as readily or as cheaply as our counterparts in the US. Alcohol for rubbing, cleaning etc. can be purchased in post-prohibition American drug stores. In the UK, if you want to get hold of quality perfume alcohol, you need a licence and the reason is not health but the duty payable to Customs and Excise. The alcohol contains additives to induce vomiting if swallowed and it has a strong, unpleasant odour which needs mellowing before use. The only companies that are excused the duty on natural grain alcohol, organic or otherwise, are medical companies which have successfully argued that product efficacy would suffer if they used perfume grade ethanol. In the UK duty is charged according to alcoholic strength of spirits and as grain alcohol is almost two and a half times the strength of most whisky, the duty payable is currently £18.78 per litre. When studying for the diploma with the Wine and Spirit Trust, the whisky module was taught by a Scot who was chief blender from a well known whisky producer. He showed us figures of how much money went each year from Scotland down to London in the form of duty. I can't recall the figures but they were astonishing.

In chapter five I present a method I have evolved for making unique fragrances for individuals and a systematic method of blending. I also kick around some ideas regarding smell from a subjective perspective. My chemistry studies at school got about as far as deliberately warming test tubes to get the contents to smoking point in order to set the fire alarm off. Recently, when I read Luca

Turin's book *The Secret of Scent*, in which he puts forward a theory of how smell works, I had to get a copy of *Chemistry for Dummies*' to try and follow his thesis. In chapter six I try and convey my thought train when blending an actual fragrance and in chapter seven I explain what I believe to be the best method of handling the raw materials.

Chapter eight contains a list of completely natural aromatic raw materials. The list represents natural materials which, in my opinion, are the most useful from a fragrance perspective. For each I mention the method and place of production but the emphasis is mostly on its use in perfumery. The origins are the most usual places that I currently source each from. It is not intended to be an exhaustive list of geographical production areas. I also add comments on points of interest, and remarks on current safety issues relevant to each material. It is important to remember that safety issues evolve and change over time. There are, for example, certain raw materials that have been used for centuries whose use is now either restricted or completely banned. Current EU legislation in this regard is more restrictive than that in America. Allergies are a common part of modern life and it has been suggested by some that our immune systems are more depleted than those of our ancestors. It also follows that the more frequently a material is used, the more likely it is to appear in statistics. I have followed the safety guidelines issued by the International Fragrance Association, which can be found at www.ifra.org

Perfume, combined with cosmetics, is the sixth largest industry on the planet measured in financial terms and yet most of us know very little about it. A friend who works for a French perfume company recently told me in jest that the perfumers are killed when they retire. How many perfumers can you name? Big brands start as family companies and as they expand, outside expertise is usually bought in. Edmond Roudnitska wrote a paper arguing for more recognition for perfumers. He argued that great perfumes are works of art, that the creativity behind them should be valued more and that there should be intellectual rights belonging to their creators. A few years ago some perfumers in France did rock the boat by wanting more recognition but the mutiny was short lived. If credit goes to the perfumer and they become a name as well as a nose the possibility of leaving the 'Firm' like many Michelin starred chefs have done becomes a dangerous possibility. The large scale commercial fragrance is all about the brand and the only personality ever associated with most perfumes will be a celebrity.

Finally, I would like to acknowledge the help and support given by so many people and extend gratitude. First and foremost, all of our customers without whom we would not have a business and in the same vein, my hardworking and loyal staff. Thanks to Fiona

Owen for accepting my commission and creating her narrative masterpiece on perfume. I thank Angela Lamond for lending her professional proofreading skills. Paul Fowler artist and picture framer extraordinaire for his eye and advice, James Crowden for pointers in publishing and Mark Savage MW for amongst other things pulling corks. Appreciation goes to Shaun Stevenson for being first among a few with whom I can share my enthusiasm for all things smelly. He also deserves gratitude for his willingness to share his knowledge, even when it stops him from working. I gassho to Eddy Street for sending me papers on psychological aspects of smell. Gratitude to Jenny Scott for support and friendship when it really mattered. Thanks go to Tanu for taking the hassle out of travelling in India, making it possible to relax into the adventure. Sara from Watershed PR I'm tempted to say your so sparky and literate but what I want to say is thank you for behaving like an old friend. Last, but not least, the two most important women in my life: my daughter Tasha for being a squidge even when getting jobbied and my partner Denise for her courage, kindness and love.

ONE

Historical Overview

The creature on our planet with the strongest sense of smell is, by a long shot, the humble moth. A Chinese emperor moth can smell a single bloom from six miles downwind. Flowers from the indolic type (jasmine, lilies, tuberose) are dependent on the moth for pollination and communicate with it by exuding their heavy, sweet scent. As moths are nocturnal, not only do these flowers produce more scent at night but their blooms lack the carotene, chlorophylls, anthocyanins and xantophylls that give other flowers colour. Their white blossoms are able to reflect light from the moon and the stars to further aid the moth to find and pollinate them. The scents from some of these white blooms even mimic the pheromones of the moth. These white, heady, sweet floral aromas provide some of the most exotic, ethereal and romantic scents. Tuberose, which was native to Mexico, was brought to Europe at the end of the 16th century. As it releases most of its heady scent at night, it is known in Malaysia as 'mistress of the night'. It is one of several oils and absolutes that are literally worth more than their weight in gold. There we have it in a nutshell – the simple reasons that humans developed an interest in fragrance and the perfume industry evolved – sex and money.

The oils and absolutes are extracted from 8 different groups of raw materials. They are: – (i) flowers, (ii) herbs, (iii) leaves and grasses, (iv) spices, (v) roots, (vi) gums and balsams, (vii) wood and (viii) citrus.

The word perfume comes from the Latin 'per', meaning 'through' and 'fummum', meaning 'smoke' which reveals the earliest uses of aromatics as incense. It doesn't require much imagination to understand the process whereby something valuable and solid was rendered ethereal by the transformative effect of fire. In its new form it could waft over the threshold into the other world, where it could be enjoyed by the ethereal beings which inhabited that realm. The incense most highly valued by the Mesopotamians was made from the aromatic cedar of Lebanon. The wood was imported by the hierarchic city-states of the Tigris and Euphrates valley.

In Egypt, records show that an expedition was made in 2800 BCE for gums and resins. However, the Egyptian word for incense appears in even earlier records. Later, another expedition was recorded in bas-reliefs on the wall of a temple near Thebes.

The accounts in Exodus (approx 1250 BCE) describing materials and their use as incense would also have been true for other cultures in the near East at that time, as their use was prevalent.

The link between Greece and those earlier cultures mentioned above can be found on Crete and Cyprus. Both inscriptions, Linear A and Linear B, at Knossos have now been deciphered. It was in these two languages that records and inventories were kept at Knossos. These records show that the Cretans had aromatic oils and that both the scent of the lily and that of a hybrid rose were popular. This early flowering in the cradle of European civilisation was cut short by destructive invading tribes. Later, when Greek culture emerged on the mainland, both Athens and Corinth were doing brisk business in aromatics by the seventh century BCE. Incense on municipal altars began to replace burnt offerings of animal sacrifices.

The Etruscans brought a civilising influence to early Roman culture, which adopted their use of perfumes. Plautus records the importation of incense from Arabia by the second century BCE.

The Arab contribution was huge. The camel was domesticated circa 500 BCE, making desert trading possible. Frankincense and myrrh from the Arabian Peninsula, along with traded goods from China, were taken to Alexandria, establishing a regular trade route. It may have been the Dark Ages in Europe but the 'lost' arts and sciences were not lost in the East. This fact was curiously absent from the history syllabus at Cheltenham Grammar School; at least it was when I was there. It was through Islam that antiquity became linked to the modern world. As Islam spread, it drew in the learning and technology of the Greco-Roman world and spread it across vast areas of Asia, Northern Africa and southern Europe. It was the Arab technologists who made improvements to distillation equipment and were able to make glass that could withstand the high temperatures necessary for quality extraction of essential oils. It was also through Islam that the West came into contact with India and China.

India possesses a wide range of climatic zones which give rise to the growing conditions necessary for a vast range of aromatic plants. Their religious traditions not only encouraged bathing but also the use of aromatic oils. From China, the West was introduced to musk and citrus fruits – Seville oranges (therefore neroli bigarade and petitgrain), tangerines, kumquats and probably lemons.

Trade delegations and Buddhist monks travelled from China to Japan, taking with them aspects of Chinese culture. Much of Japanese culture originated in China but the Japanese also made it their own by applying their highly developed sense of aesthetic. Incense making evolved into an art form and a scent-meditation game called koh-do evolved. It became fashionable to carry perfumes in inros (a small ornamented box hung from the waist sash of a kimono) and olfaction was cultivated as part of civilised life.

The Renaissance signalled the end of the so-called Dark Ages in Europe. The emergence of this new 'world' was largely characterised by technical studies. Distillation techniques had been developed and improved by generations of Arab and Chinese alchemists but in about 1200 a monumental breakthrough occurred in Southern Europe with the discovery of the secret of alcohol.

Most of Europe had inherited a theology that denigrated the body but this was one of the attitudes that the Renaissance was going to challenge. Alexandrian culture, being largely a blend of Egyptian and Hellenistic, was much kinder to 'brother donkey'. Neo-Platonists of the Academy of the Medici in Florence had begun preaching the nobility of the human condition and this attitude was embraced by Italian intellectuals and later absorbed by the French. Personal grooming began to be not only acceptable but fashionable. The stage was set for the emergence of the modern perfumery trade.

Since the domestication of the camel, the Arabs were middlemen in traded goods between Europe and the Far East. The European desire to trade direct with the Orient had been stimulated by mysterious tales of Marco Polo's voyages and of exotic spice producing islands, bizarre marketplaces and coffers of untold wealth. Venice enjoyed the best trading relationship with the Arabs and it was for this reason alone that the perfume industry developed in Italy. However, Portuguese nautical acumen was about to spoil the party. Vasco De Gama set sail from Lisbon and headed south, then east, before arriving in Calcutta on May 20 1498. He had successfully sailed round Africa, thereby connecting the Atlantic with the Orient. His ship returned to Lisbon laden with benzoin, cinnamon, ginger, pepper and cloves. Once the news reached Venice their stock exchange took a tumble and the Italians dispatched a fleet to take on the Portuguese in the Indian Ocean. Portuguese men of war against gondolas? Indian Ocean? Melting Cornettos? I think not. The decisive Portuguese victory facilitated a shift in the centre of the perfume industry from the Mediterranean to the Atlantic where it has remained to this day.

Further battles over natural resources followed. Trading companies and Empires emerged as the Dutch, the English and the

French all wanted their share of the riches to be had from the Orient, along with the Portuguese. The social and economic situation in much of Europe now favoured the emergence of the modern perfume trade. Firstly, large amounts of wealth were generated by the new class of merchants who also provided copious quantities of aromatic raw materials from distant, exotic locations. Further improvements in glass making became possible with higher firing temperatures when charcoal was replaced for smelting by coal and coke.

Kid gloves from Grasse had been fashionable with European nobility for centuries. It is rumoured that the first Queen Elizabeth had 1,200 pairs. The hides were cured using urine and the smell of the urine was masked by using civet. Grasse was well placed to take advantage of its position and become a link between the new Atlantic trade and the earlier Mediterranean cultures of Italy and the Levant. During the reign of Louis XIV interest in perfume became huge and this ensured both the prevalence of France and Grasse in the perfume industry, which was about to explode.

During the French Revolution, most Aristocrats became more cost-conscious and less extravagant than usual, so it would be fairly safe to assume that sales of luxury items, including perfume, were down in the new democracy. However, the revolution went to Napoleon's head and he became Emperor. As Emperor, he was hugely influential and not only did he have a considerable interest in perfume himself but he was also willing to support talent over nobility of birth. This culture was very supportive of both entrepreneurs and technologists.

There are many apocryphal stories about Napoleon's relationship with smell and perfume. He is supposed to have written to Josephine, 'I'll be back in one month – don't wash.' He is also supposed to have liked neroli on her but not musk. The aristocratic Josephine became a fashion icon and Napoleon's second wife, Eugenie, had a strong sense of style and love of ornamentation. These two ladies influenced fashion in France just as much as they would have done had they been royals. It is said that good musk will last for three centuries. Apparently, when Napoleon dumped Josephine, a parting gift from her was to liberally sprinkle musk all over his apartment.

Further scientific progress towards the end of the 19th Century led to the first aroma chemicals (aldehydes) and technical developments in glass making led to mass production. The stage was now set for La Belle Époque and the emergence of the bottle as art form.

As far as we can gather, the early perfumes were probably quite simple affairs. The notion of grouping different constituents by their molecular weight (top, middle and base notes) and harnessing them in layers to increase interest and tenacity did not evolve until the end of the 19th century. Prior to this, there is much evidence to suggest that single note fragrances were the most usual kind. However, the emphasis was definitely on the fragrance rather than the container and prior to adequate glass manufacturing techniques it was the silversmith who provided the containers for those wealthy enough to afford them.

Before the advent of the railways, European spa resorts were the preserve of the nobility and a few wealthy industrialists. The Industrial Revolution created new working places peopled by those no longer dependent on the land for subsistence. As many new industries developed, new wealth trickled down to some extent and a growing number enjoyed disposable income. Railway travel was relatively cheap and travelling great distances was much more viable than it had been by horse. Travel became more accessible to lower income groups and along with the spa resorts, seaside resorts emerged and people began travelling as a form of leisure activity. Tourists were keen to carry home proof of their exploits and they were not to be disappointed by the range of knick-knacks soon to be on offer. Of interest to us is the souvenir bottle. These bottles were sold empty, usually quite small, made of glass and with a hand painted vignette of their chosen destination on the lid. They were, and still are, collectable.

What concerns us here is a shift in emphasis from the contents of the bottle onto the bottle itself. Bottles became of increasing importance to the newly emerging perfume houses. Numbered limited edition bottles, which had been designed by well-known artists, became a marketing tool. A small number of dedicated companies, notably Lalique and Baccarat, specialised in making beautiful bottles.

A few years later, another shift was going to happen and one that has stuck to this day. It came about as a consequence of changing social conditions and sophisticated modern marketing techniques. We may as well start with James Dean and Elvis Presley and the emergence of the teenager as a separate social group with disposable income. Prior to this, there had been heart throbs like Douglas Fairbanks, Rudolph Valentino and Attila the Hun but something very significant in the social fabric of European-influenced societies was about to change. Along with the emergence of the teenager came relativism (as opposed to some kind of objective value system) and it is this, perhaps more than any other single factor, that creates the tsunami which celebrities surf. It has become possible to be famous just for being famous.

During a visit to Kenya I came into contact with the Samburu tribe and had many conversations with a very handsome and noble young warrior called Lamekyeo. His English was excellent and he had read widely including, I'm afraid, Jeffrey Archer. Though the tribal lifestyle was going through some necessary changes to negotiate survival in the modern world, the social structures which had preserved a traditional lifestyle for centuries were still clearly visible. Personal roles were completely subordinate to the survival of the tribe. At the time of first menstruation an adolescent girl would be isolated from all but her mother and aunts. She spent much time alone to ponder the meaning of becoming a woman and a giver of life. Adolescent boys had to undertake a perilous journey to a distant mountain armed only with a spear. A token had to be collected from the mountain to prove to the elders that the journey had been completed. Not all the boys made it back. Those that did, returned as men, were able to take a wife and become warriors. The warriors' job was primarily to protect the tribe and the tribe's cattle from the perils of the bush (not Dubya). When they became too old to be warriors or bear children they became elders and custodians of the traditions for the next generation. The elders told Lamekyeo that he thought too much and I must confess to sending him some books on my return to England.

In the land of plenty authentic initiations are hard to find and even harder are elders with real wisdom. So we play the mating game and fabricate identities. I read an article a while ago about the number of Elvis Presley imitators compared with how many there were when Elvis was alive. Apparently, if we continue the trend we will reach a point in about 20 years where half the people on the planet will be dressed as Elvis; the other half, by then, will be obese.

Psychologically speaking, in Western cultures adolescence is characterised by narcissism and an unshakeable belief in how special one is. Psychological dependency on the parents is replaced by identifying with a tribal group (Teddy boys, Goths, Mods, football team etc.); this is, of course, a necessary part of separating from parents and the beginning of the maturation process and as long as one doesn't get stuck with the tribe can facilitate individuation and psychological autonomy later in life. The fact that most people do get stuck is the chink through which the marketing men can hook us. The shift that I'm talking about is one away from the contents of the bottle altogether and onto the dream showing now in all the glossies.

According to Luca Turin in his recent book, *The Secret of Scent*, just 3% of the money we pay for a mainstream fragrance pays for the smell content; the other 97% is the bill for selling us the dream (see page 13). When you watch fragrance commercials on television, notice how they don't tell you about what's in the bottle. We are encouraged to believe that instead of riding round the world on a Triumph, that was actually a BMW, we just need to splash some of this on. Do you never want to sleep alone again? Well, honey, then buy this and instantly achieve the lifestyle alluded to in this picture.

Of course, if you're really, really, really rich then shopping to make yourself feel really, really, really special becomes an art form and you develop a curious kind of co-dependency on the illusionists that you need to help you believe that you are, oh, so very special. New age pop psychology would have me believe that we are all special but surely that would make us all ordinary. What a relief. If, however, ordinary is not enough, don't worry – help is at hand. A fragrance called V1 starts from £65,000 for a small bottle. Alternatively, another bottle has just gone on sale in a Manchester department store for over £100,000. Presumably, planning permission for a stall outside a footballer's house was not forthcoming.

Today, mass marketing, opportunism and a myriad of celebrity scents sporting notes of candyfloss, cup cakes and bubble gum have led to a diminution of quality and kudos. I believe that there is the beginning of a modern movement in more authentic perfumery, which is gaining ground. It is partly because of a wider change in perception, which prefers 'natural' but it is also a search for the experience and appreciation of beauty. The popularity of essential oils over the last 25 years has introduced many people to the beauty of nature via the sense of smell. There are, of course, fashions in smell and as Turin points out, most successful fragrances are copies of another successful fragrance. The global market is dominated by six large companies that are behind all the major brands. This fact means that change will be slow. I concur fully with Roudnitska's statement that quality in perfume (or any other endeavour) is entirely dependent upon an educated consumer.

TWO

Sourcing Natural Raw Materials

Quality control of essential oils and absolutes is the single most important issue for any reputable company trading in natural aromatics. Every company likes to make claims about the purity of their oils, from the largest right down to the one-man band operating out of mom's kitchen. These claims would only be meaningful if other companies were claiming to sell oils that are cheap rubbish. Marketing information has led to some confusion about the reliability of certain tests. It is an uncomfortable truth that if there was a reliable test for the purity of essential oils, the market would not be flooded with low quality adulterated 'soups' passing themselves off as genuine. I shall explain why.

The first step in quality control is to define what 'quality' is. Secondly, in relation to this definition of quality we need to decide upon parameters and thirdly, we must find a way to measure data in relation to the defined parameters. Let us look in turn at each of these.

- ***Quality***: Essential oils, like all natural products, will vary from one year to another. In some cases, like geranium, there can be extreme variations in oil extracted from plants growing in different parts of the same field. It is also true that there are differences from one year to another. The plant, the soil, the weather and the microclimate all affect the odour profile and the constituents of an essential oil.

The pharmaceutical industry in the UK laid down some standards for commonly used oils, which they called B.P. (British Pharmacopoeia). A method of testing was also prescribed to ascertain if an essential oil met the criteria. The test involved heating a sample of oil to a certain temperature for a period of time, causing much of it to evaporate and measuring the residue. Eucalyptus, peppermint and clove are still sold in the UK as B.P. qualities. Since these tests were devised, extraction technology has evolved to the extent that modern pure oils will not pass these tests. There are recipes that are used to make up oils which will pass B.P. standards and these involve blending with 'nature identical' chemicals. Many B.P. qualities are typically only 80% essential oil and contrary to what many pharmacists believe, they are very low quality in comparison with other well-sourced oils of the same type.

Another way of trying to define quality is a characteristic odour profile. Bergamot oil from Sicily is a completely different animal than bergamot from the Ivory Coast – so do we have one standard for both, or two different standards for bergamot? At present, international standards do not recognize the origin of an essential oil as a factor. Due to the difficulties already described, quality parameters for essential oils are very wide. It follows that the wider the parameters are, the more scope there will be for adulteration in the service of profit.

Lavender is a Mediterranean species and as such it needs hot sun and well-drained soil. If lavender oil doesn't get enough sun, the camphor content in the oil remains too high and the floral characteristics do not develop. Conversely, peppermint likes moisture and grows well in damp conditions. I believe that climate should be taken into account when defining an oil's characteristic odour.

I propose the following definition of characteristic odour:-

1. The plant must be the mother species (as opposed to an interspecific cross, clone or hybrid).
2. The plant must be grown in an area where the species is indigenous.
3. The oil must be 100% extracted from the named botanical species.
4. The extraction technology should remove the complete oil rather than a fraction and do so without 'burning' it.

- ***Parameters***: Once we have an oil sample that we believe exhibits the characteristic odour we can use gas chromatography to analyse the constituents. This form of analysis is routinely used in the industry in an attempt to remove subjectivity. However, the large users of essential oils want product repeatability so that their products are the same every year. This means that oils are frequently adjusted to conform to a company's criteria for a certain product. In many cases, cost is the overriding factor.

- ***Measuring Data***: Essential oils and absolutes are volatile, which means that they have a tendency to vaporise. Analysis by gas chromatography produces a trace, which shows the order in which the constituents vaporise and the quantity of each constituent expressed as a percentage. For example, cineole and terpinen-4-ol in Tea Tree will always show up in the same place on the time axis of the graph. The trace for good tea tree oil will always show a similar pattern. Some oils have so many constituents (rose has over 400) that many of them do not even have names but are referred to simply by co-ordinates (time and % quantity) on the trace. Many oils have constituents in common but the proportions differ which is why they have different odours. (Please see appendix for example of gas chromatography trace and analysis).

A gas chromatography trace will tell us the quantity of each constituents but it cannot tell us whether the oil is pure or not. Supposing when tea tree oil is being distilled some eucalyptus accidentally fell into the still. Unlikely as this may seem, it is worth remembering that most tea tree oil production happens in Australia where everything is upside down. The resulting oil will be higher in 1.8 cineole (quality eucalyptus is at least 80% 1.8 cineole). An analysis by gas chromatography will tell us how much cineole is in the oil but it will not tell us that the source of some of the 1.8 cineole was eucalyptus. Spanish rosemary is routinely distilled with camphor wood to make a more economic distillation. This is surprising, as Spain isn't even sideways, let alone upside down.

The situation is made even more complex by the fact that so many of these constituents are available as natural isolates or aroma chemicals.

I believe that the best method for obtaining pure high grade essential oils is based on the quality of relationship that we have with our suppliers. It is honestly that simple. After over twenty years in the business one should get to know who can and who cannot be trusted. Further, elective affinities mean that the rogues and the more honest guys tend not to hang out in the same groups.

Shortly after the lavender harvest I will obtain perhaps as many as twenty samples. I will be looking for a strong floral character with herbaceous undertones and very low 1.8 cineole. I would also expect it to be tenacious on a smelling strip. When I have decided on which I prefer, I will get details about the price and the quantity available. The producer will also send me an analysis. When I have the sample analysed I expect the results to be the same as those sent by the producer. If they are different I buy my oil from someone else. After doing this for over twenty years we know whom we can trust.

Handling and Storage

As oil arrives at a warehouse, inspection should be made immediately to make sure that the quality is the same as the sample. Each approved batch is then moved into an oil store which is secure, dark, and consistently cool. Certain absolutes are kept in a fridge. The quantity of oil we buy is determined by the shelf life and the amount we sell. Some oils, like patchouli, vetivert and sandalwood improve with age whilst others deteriorate. Lemon, for example, has a tendency to oxidise so we have regular deliveries of smaller amounts which we bottle immediately so that it is not sitting around in a drum half full of oxygen. Records are kept of delivery dates, batches and production schedules to ensure appropriate stock rotation. Once bottled, our oils are boxed and stored in a cool warehouse ready for dispatch.

Quality should be top of the list for any serious company genuinely interested in its reputation. The next most important issue is cost and that is nearly always related to volume. In terms of importing oils and absolutes directly it is simply not worth bothering for small quantities: the fixed costs are just too high to make it worthwhile. This is even more the case today due to post 9/11 security charges. The charges for the necessary paperwork by the freight forwarding companies are virtually the same, whether a single kilo or a tonne is being imported. Pro rata freight charges become much more reasonable with larger volumes in single shipments.

There is a well-established network of companies that move very large quantities of certain oils around the globe. As a relatively small essential oil company, we can buy 50 kg of Paraguayan petitgrain oil much more cheaply from someone who imports it by the tonne rather than going direct ourselves. For some of the more precious oils it may be worth going directly to a producer. However, good producers may be difficult to find, especially when there may be communication problems and language difficulties. A certain patchouli producer in Indonesia, for example, takes three weeks to answer a fax.

Recently, I was trying to find a trading partner in India to buy some quite rare and expensive absolutes. Anyone who has travelled in that completely wonderful, but sometimes maddening, land will know that if one is trying to buy genuine pashmina then many traders will have no compunction in selling you an army blanket if they can get away with it.

I established fax and email contact with a particular producer which boasts several companies trading under different names. I opened with some technical gambits that were batted with ease. I got more technical, not because I was being pretentious but because I wanted to discover if they were genuine producers. I even got a close friend living in Kashmir, with whom I have travelled many times in India, to give them a call and see if he could suss them out. His feedback suggested that they certainly knew their onions and seemed genuine. I decided to buy some samples costing about £165, making it quite clear that if the materials were genuine and they were a reliable supplier then potentially I could be spending quite large amounts on a monthly basis. I was given a tracking number for my parcel of samples and after a few days went on line to see where it was. Inadvertently, they had given me the wrong number so I was able to see that quite a large parcel was on its way to Moscow.

When my parcel did arrive, I ripped it apart with all the enthusiasm of a spaniel at Christmas. To my disappointment, the samples were complete junk and I had been made to wear a topee. I should explain here that this expression is Delhi street slang. The origination of the phrase goes back to a time when important people used to wear large hats called topees, the more important the larger the topee. Of course, to a casual observer someone wearing a very large hat with an air of self-importance might look a complete clown. The Hindi phrase (topee panana charta eh?) translates as 'Are you trying to make me wear a topee?' So getting a topee is getting ripped off.

I contacted the company in question and received an immediate refund on my credit card. They knew darn well what they had done, hence the speed of the refund. Thankfully, now that *White Tiger* (Booker prize winning novel revealing level of corruption in India written by a native) has been published, I can say without fear of contradiction that this kind of opportunism in India is rife. It is probably the biggest single factor preventing wealth from trickling down.

Thirty years ago only imps, pimps and banjo players used essential oils and they were quite hard to get hold of in retail quantities. As the market grew with the explosion of aromatherapy, middle men traders emerged. Most of these guys had worked previously for various perfume houses and because of this had, in some cases, quite deep knowledge about the oils themselves. The early aromatherapy trainings focused almost entirely upon the assumed therapeutic uses of the oils rather than looking at the oils themselves in detail. Because of this disparity, some of these traders assumed almost Guru-like authority amongst aromatherapists. Not surprisingly, like the best Gurus some of them abused their position.

By and large, the job of a perfume house is to work to a brief supplied by their customers. This invariably involves product repeatability and price stability. The highly trained chemists have at their disposal an arsenal of synthetic and natural raw materials which can be skilfully blended to achieve the desired effect and price. Even if these middle men traders did not have this knowledge themselves they had access to those that did. There is absolutely nothing wrong with this, as it would be quite pointless to use a high grade of rose otto for a mass produced soap, or cold pressed Sicilian lemon oil in toilet bleach. However, what is wrong is for somebody to sell one thing and knowingly call it another.

THREE

Sandalwood

Aqua Oleum has been sourcing sandalwood oil from the only genuinely sustainable source that we know of. It is not true, as has been suggested, that sandalwood is an endangered species. It is only an endangered species in parts of India. There are huge areas of forest containing sandalwood trees in both Laos and Cambodia but there is no timber or oil production because the terrain is too hostile and, for the present at least, production would be uneconomic. The three main areas which produce sandalwood oil have been India, Indonesia and New Caledonia. There are also small productions from other sources e.g. Australia and Fiji.

1. India – the main producer for years of the genuine oil from *Santalum Album*. The wood has long been in very high demand for religious statues, prayer beads and incense as well as for oil.

There have been attempts by the government at sustainability but the producers have undermined these. As the price for the oil has increased, so has the incentive for bucking the system. Adulteration is prolific. The mainland genuine species should be at least 30 or 40 years old before it is used for oil production – many are used younger. Even with intensive planting and re-planting of young trees, it would take many years before India became sustainable. Logs are being imported from Australia of a non-sandalwood species called *Eucaria Spicata* and these are being used in so-called sandalwood production. We have recently been offered Indian sandalwood and one sample which was tested contained 40% Spicata. This particular sample came from a reliable source, which shows how endemic the problem is.

2. Indonesia – since the civil war the infrastructure has seriously deteriorated. East Timor, by far the main producer, is now independent. There are two factories: one barely functions, possibly due to it being wrecked by the Indonesian authorities before they left; the other is funded by a multi-national fragrance company, which has become very reluctant to provide any more money due to the overall situation. Production has become very spasmodic – only three parcels were available last year (2007). The East Timor government has more pressing problems than sandalwood and is focussed on aid, hospitals and food programmes.

3. New Caledonia – a group of Islands in the South Pacific. Most were part of the French colonies but not all were inhabited by Europeans. We source our oil from an Island called Vanuatu, which used to be a British colony. The island has been producing sandalwood for over 200 years on a small scale. Natural regeneration has compensated for any production over the last 20 years. Sandalwood requires a host plant (like mistletoe) in order to grow. As they develop roots, the seedlings tap into the root system of the host plant in order to get nutrients. Once the sandalwood tree is established it can survive even if the host plant dies. The seeds are very hardy and if cleared areas are left, rainfall can precipitate regeneration from naturally scattered seeds.

The government has been controlling production for the last ten years. They have seen what had happened on neighbouring French Islands – namely, using up all the trees over decades without replanting. As the demand grew for the oil younger and younger trees were taken, eventually destroying the industry. Another factor has been the decline of the local fishing industry, which has increased the need to develop the sandalwood production. Sandalwood production is now strictly controlled on Vanuatu. The government issues licenses, which go to auction. Initially, only two companies were allowed to bid for these licenses. The licenses designate areas where production is allowed – individual, mature trees are marked by the government department so thinning is controlled, as is replanting. Felling is only allowed to take place in August, which combined with the Island location makes enforcement easy. The Islanders appreciate the importance of sustainability and the government has also introduced a scheme whereby they give a small sandalwood tree on a host plant to anyone who wants to plant one on their allotment. These trees can then be sold at maturity forming a mini-pension. The indigenous species is *Santalum Austrocaledonicum*, which is a genuine subspecies. As an Island species it grows more quickly than mainland varieties and can be used after fifteen years. The area of coverage by sandalwood trees on the island has now increased from its original natural size. The host plants that are used also produce nuts and oil for fuel and lubricants. The benefits and income from the production stay on the island.

The initial trials for oil production produced some good quality samples. However, Taiwan had been buying the wood for some years and when offered oil, accepted. The jump in production necessary to supply Taiwan led to a diminution of quality. Our oil is now rectified, which means it is distilled a second time and topped and tailed. The second distillation has a refining effect and removes any mal odours. Traditionally, the first oil out of the still is called the 'top' and the last oil at the end of the distillation is called the 'tail'. The rectification process reduces the overall yield by approximately 25%.

The company which supplies our oil is also funding some research. Sandalwood trees have been used locally in skin care preparations and different properties have been observed from different trees. Locally, the trees are known as black or white – though despite being the same colour the names have come down through history. It is thought that this is to do with the properties observed in the oil. One suggestion is that there may be male and female trees.

In terms of quality, good Indian oil, with its characteristic deep, warm, soft, balsamic, sweet-woody scent, is the benchmark. However, this quality from India is now extremely rare for reasons outlined above. It is still available but at a price. The Indonesian production, despite being obtained from the genuine species, has to our mind always lacked the warmth and softness of the Indian material; it can also have mild pithy and some smoky notes.

The most effective way of converting sandalwood logs into money is through selling the oil. However, the best oil comes from the roots and the base of the trunk. The remaining sections have traditionally been used for religious statues, prayer beads and incense. There are some log companies operating legally which have supplied sandalwood to Taiwan, Singapore and India for decades. Plenty of logs from Vanuatu can be seen at distilleries in the Mysore area. In fact, the Indians have started buying more of these logs and as the government on Vanuatu restrict the amount available each year the price has just jumped by 50% (October 2008). Happily, as it is being currently managed it is sustainable and is being cultivated by Islanders for themselves. Mysore sandalwood will always command a premium price as it is second to none in quality. It therefore follows that oil being passed off as genuine Mysore sandalwood will potentially command the same price.

Australian sandalwood oil from *Eucaria Spicata* will become very restricted. An Australian producer has been taken over and all normal supplies have been put on hold. The new owner has negotiated with 5 big fragrance houses to supply them with their sandalwood. In round figures the 5 fragrance houses need between 15 and 16 tons a year, whereas Australian production is 12 tons per year. It looks like the price of the Australian oil could possibly double soon. New Caledonia usually looks towards Australia rather than India to set their prices so sharp increases can be expected. Indian material will certainly continue rising in price. We imagine that as prices increase, as they have been doing for some time, qualities, especially at the retail end, will continue to deteriorate. My worry is that in the long term fewer people will know just how wonderful authentic Mysore oil is. People are accustomed to paying high prices for absolutes, but to do so for a steam distilled oil a psychological hurdle needs to be jumped. Those of us who have jumped would do well to squirrel some away. Those involved in the authentic perfume trade realise how thoroughly versatile and useful this oil is. It is certainly on a par with rose maroc. The good news is that sandalwood improves with age and will keep for many decades if stored properly.

On a recent trip to India I discovered the truth behind some of the rumours about sandalwood oil production and export. Anyone who has travelled off piste in India will be aware to what extent local mafia and dacoits have their fingers in the pie. In the Mysore area there was a very famous and powerful dacoit called Veerappan. Apparently, he had an interest in much of the Mysore sandalwood oil production. Further, on a daily basis perhaps 200 to 300 tourists venture into the Mysore jungle, mostly to watch wildlife. There were a number of kidnappings and ransom demands involving some quite well-known Indians taken as hostages of Mr Veerappan. On one occasion he held an Indian film star for 108 days. In an attempt to cut his funding at source the Indian government banned both the export of sandalwood and sandalwood oil. However, the plan backfired because they succeeded in creating a black market with the corresponding price rises. He is reputed to have smuggled $22 m US worth of sandalwood. He was wanted for over 100 murders and has evaded the police for many years, earning him a notorious reputation.

An elite Indian army squad were sent into the jungle to try and track down our friend. They came across an enormous store of Mysore sandalwood logs. It was reported to have been the largest haul ever seen and represented about 50% of all available at that time. The Mysore jungle in places is very thick and inaccessible so removing these logs naturally presented a problem. Traditionally, elephants would have been used for such a task: sadly, another natural resource not ignored by Mr. Pan, who was reputed to have smuggled nearly $3 m US of ivory. The official story is that as the logistics of removal were insurmountable, the Army exercised their right of pyromania. Now maybe I'm being cynical, but I cannot imagine a large pile of highly valuable logs, in quite an inaccessible and discrete store in thick jungle in

India, just being torched. The wonder of India is the mystery.

Many years ago I was suspicious about the quality of some sandalwood oil that I had bought from one of my regular suppliers. I had the oil independently tested and my suspicions were confirmed. I requested and received an analysis from the supplier. Needless to say, it bore no relation to the results that I had obtained. My relationship with this supplier was terminated. Some years later the consumer Magazine 'Which' launched an independent enquiry into the quality of essential oils being offered by different retail outlets. Sandalwood oil being sold in a small chain of shops was taken for analysis; the results showed that it contained no sandalwood oil at all. The person who owned these shops had to carry the can but the real culprit was the supplier who got off scot-free. It is worth remembering that good conmen are credible and that some shops may stock over 2,000 items, making specialist product knowledge across such a wide range unrealistically demanding. After several more misdemeanours the person in question was expelled from a trade association and has since acquired a company which remains a member of that same association.

I remember hearing about a company wishing to import sandalwood directly from India. They made contact with the supplier, samples were sent and approved and drums ordered. When the drums arrived in the UK it was winter. The top was removed from each drum and a sample drawn and quality approved. However, sometime later when someone went to move the drums they noticed something peculiar about the feel of the drum. Apparently, about 70% of the contents were coconut oil, which had solidified due to the cold weather. The 30% of sandalwood which had not solidified floated above the coconut oil, creating the impression of pukka gear. Complaints were made and the initial response from the Indians was, 'Well you approved the sample.' Once it had been explained to them that the name of their company would be circulated around many companies in the industry, they relented and made good.

Meanwhile, one of our middlemen friends referred to above has so alienated certain suppliers that they refuse to deal with him. One of the alienated suppliers is a large citrus player in the UK and another one of the largest volume suppliers of both lavender and lavendin in the UK. Periodically, the lavender supplier gets a call from a broker who asks what the current spot rates are for lavender and lavendin. Every time that they receive this phone call they know that the person they have refused to deal with is behind it and he is fishing to find out how to undercut other suppliers. Rates are hiked appropriately.

FOUR

Natural and Synthetic

Natural ingredients available to the modern perfumer number somewhere between 400 to 500 and are extracted from different parts of aromatic plants. This compares with about 5,000 synthetic aroma chemicals. These are either constituents that have been separated from a plant oil (isolates) or manufactured from alcohol, coal tar or other petro-chemical derivatives. We must not forget that coal and petro-chemicals started life in plant form and can also, from a broad perspective, be called natural. Think of them as well-aged ferns.

From the perspective of the perfume industry, there are several advantages to using synthetics. The most obvious one is cost. Many of the most expensive floral absolutes are so costly because the yield of oil is so low. In order to make 1kg of rose otto, for example, 10,000kgs of roses are needed. It so happens that these precious floral absolutes are also very labour intensive to harvest. Some like jasmine and tuberose must even be picked at night – usually by hand. I have never heard anyone claim that a synthetic rose or jasmine can entirely replace a natural one but judicious blending can achieve a compromise with which many are happy. It is largely a question of economics, taste and education.

At one time nylon, polyester and corfam were going to transform our lives by making us modern and fashionable. Who would not prefer silk, cotton, wool and leather assuming they could afford them and that the choice was available?

Historically, some of the best ingredients for perfume making were of animal origin – musk, ambergris, civet and castoreum being the main four. There are serious ethical issues around using any of these ingredients now, as either cruelty or slaughter is needed to produce them. In my experience all reputable companies would not use them but an unethical trade still carries on in some of them. These products give a magical 'tweak' to perfumes and can literally transform a blend from being quite interesting into something sensational. The fact that these animal derived fixatives are now available as synthetics is of major importance. There is no justification for using them today, although it remains a topic of debate whether it is possible to replicate what they brought to a perfume. I know many in the perfume trade who believe that most perfume of today is not of its former quality because these original fixatives are no longer used.

Out of interest, here is a brief summary of each.

Musk

Musk is produced by a small deer (*Moschus mochiferus*), which is native to Western China and Tibet. The stag has a small pouch just in front of the abdomen, which gives off sexual signals by releasing the prized aroma. It is about the size of a walnut and can be removed without 'harming' the donor. The sac is dried before being offered for sale. The material removed from these sacs is in the form of grains, which are so concentrated as to be putrid before dilution, after which it becomes extremely pleasant and sweet.

Genuine musk can still be found but it is not used much because of its cost. It is also quite rightly considered unethical. There are apparently musk farms in China as well as many synthetic substitutes.

Ambergris

Produced by the sperm whale (*Physeter catodon*). This large mammal feeds on cuttlefish, which contain a porous central bone as sold in pet shops for sharpening the beaks of birds. As this bone is indigestible and abrasive, it irritates the stomach lining of the whale. The whale secretes ambergris to protect itself from the irritation. Sometimes the whale will cough up these aromatic lumps and they may float around for months being tossed by the sea and warmed by the sun. A process which mellows, softens and adds complexity to the aroma. Lumps of ambergris could be trapped in a fisherman's net or washed up on a beach. Whaling ships would also find the substance when a whale was cut open, providing the Captain with a welcome perk which could be sold for large sums. When fresh, it is oily and repugnant. There are stories of sailors vomiting after smelling it. Ambergris was one of the most valuable commodities in the ancient world and aged ambergris found by beachcombers or caught in nets was more valuable than the fresh material.

Most common in the Indian Ocean, it became known to the Arabs who appreciated its sweet odour and its fixative properties. Most commonly, the oily lumps weigh a pound or two but have been found weighing up to seventy pounds or even more. Its fragrance is very persistent and it is said will last for three centuries. Ten different types have been identified as coming from different geographical areas and classified according to colour and aroma.

The growing scarcity, cost and concern about killing whales have all contributed to its demise. Aged ambergris has a similar aroma to labdanum and there are also synthetic substitutes.

Civet

Civet is a glandular secretion of a cat (*Viverra civetta*), which is native to East Africa. A fatty substance forms by the genitalia of both sexes and can be removed twice a week from mature cats. Like most fixatives it has a revolting fecal odour that becomes pleasant with magical fixing properties once diluted. There are civet farms in Ethiopia where the cats, which only grow as big as four feet in length, are kept in cages. As it is secreted by both genders, it probably has a role in marking territory as well as sending sexual signals. This view is supported by the fact that when the cats are made aggressive they produce more civet. I have heard stories of these cats being prodded with sharpened sticks to stimulate the production.

There have been attempts to farm the cats elsewhere but Africa remains the main source. The key constituent 'civetone' is now made synthetically. Historically, civet has been the most important of all the animal fixatives and could be previously found in most of the top quality perfumes.

The civet cat is also renowned for the transformative effect it can have upon the coffee bean. The cat picks and swallows individual beans which pass through the digestive tract and are excreted whole. These beans, when dried and roasted, make the most sublime coffee. I personally have never tried it but someone I know who is a coffee afficionado had three double espressos made from the beans in rapid succession. He waited, expecting the usual kick after such indulgence and was surprised when none came. He also said that it was the best coffee he had tried in his entire life. There have been attempts to produce civet coffee from cats in captivity but farmers were unable to replicate the ability of the cat to select individual coffee beans appropriately.

Castoreum

Both sexes of a beaver (*Castor faber*) found in Russia and Canada secrete this substance into two abdominal sacs. It is also known as beaver musk or oil and castor. It was used as a diluent in wine and favoured for particularly heavy oriental type fragrances. Being rare and costly, it has gone out of fashion but is imitated in some modern fragrances.

Most fragrances made today use a high proportion of synthetic ingredients. If all fragrances attempted to be natural there would simply not be enough natural raw materials to make this a reality. There are already environmental issues around illegally felled and smuggled logs along a trail from

East Africa through parts of the Arab world to Asia. Rather than the emergence of strongly polarised natural and synthetic camps, I would rather that we see ourselves as being part of the same industry. That does not mean that we cannot have preferences or differences, or that each camp doesn't have issues that need addressing. Big business can behave badly and can mislead to turn a profit for the shareholders but there are many small companies that are unethical, either by default through ignorance (lack of training), or blatantly making claims that cannot be substantiated (about origin and grade of raw material, organic status etc). To quote a friend, 'honesty, originality and skill have always been in shorter supply than greed, imitation and stupidity.'

Many people would be shocked to discover that it is perfectly legal to say that a fragrance has notes of jasmine when it actually doesn't contain any jasmine whatsoever. The blend of chemicals that attempt to replicate the odour profile of jasmine are simply referred to as jasmine in promotional literature and advertisements but need only appear as 'parfum' in the listing of ingredients.

I have worked commercially with natural aromatic raw materials for just over twenty years. This has given me some understanding of their properties but I am still learning every day and hope I continue to do so. My early attempt to make fragrances fell short and much experimentation was needed to get me to the point where I felt confident and able to produce something I could be proud of. Due to the nature of my work, I had privileged access to natural aromatic raw materials and I also had my love of cooking and my knowledge of wine to inform me.

I was very used to blending essential oils with other oil based products but they behaved completely differently when blended in alcohol. I also discovered by using only naturals that only certain things work while others didn't. I understood from my wine studies that structure was needed to show the fruit at its best. In wine, the structure is provided by acidity and tannin. The sweetest desert wine needs to be high in acidity otherwise it becomes like a putrid, overripe melon. A novice taster may not notice the acidity because the sugar is more immediately obvious but remove the acidity and the wine is virtually undrinkable. In Turin's book, *The Secret of Scent*, he quotes Rene Laruelle: 'synthetics are the bones of fragrance, naturals are the flesh'. I believe that there is an optimum balance needed between these two to achieve a beautiful, beguiling fragrance that has enough tenacity and interest to perform well. The modern trend for cheap synthetic aromatics has gone too far for those of us who demand real pleasure from our fragrances. I suspect that it is difficult to get someone who is planted firmly in the 'naturals' camp to admit the limitations of that approach.

My own experience tells me that the best possible outcome is achieved by a very high proportion of naturals and a very small amount of synthetic fragrance compounds. Naturals bring complexity, delicacy, subtlety and surprise but can lack tenacity and structure. I believe this was the combination that was used when the greatest perfumes of all were created. Modern sensibility limits the use of the animal fixatives but in every other respect we are free to employ this winning combination.

In order to try to surmount this last issue, I contacted a colleague and was fortunate enough to be allowed to smell authentic samples of musk, civet and ambergris. I must point out that these materials are not being used by my colleague but as he has spent his life in the perfume industry, he has retained samples for reference.

So how was it for me? Ambergris was definitely reminiscent of the ocean. It was much more delicate than seaweed absolute but it had warmth, so also reminded me of oak moss with a hint of labdanum, like smoky vanilla. Musk grains smelt of sex and took me back to Africa. I made a vain attempt to escape the millennium by going into the bush in Kenya. At the time of my visit, elephants were on heat and exuded a musky substance from pores just behind their ears. I could quite often detect this smell twenty minutes before seeing the offending elephant. It was precisely this which I was reminded of by the musk.

Some people, who are planted firmly in the 'natural' camp, can fall into the error of believing that natural is synonymous with safe. At worst this can lead to a closed minded tendency to demonise anything that is not 'natural'. Mild allergic reactions to many aldehydic chemicals are well documented, as are some more dangerous reactions to common ingredients in mass produced perfumes and cosmetics. Let us not forget that there are also some serious issues around toxicity and photosensitivity with natural oils, not just synthetics.

Mild allergic reactions to orange oil are not that uncommon. Inhalation can cause light wheezing and direct contact with the skin can cause mild inflammation. Orange oil remains an ingredient in many household products from floor cleaners to soft drinks. Bergamot oil needs the furancoumarin removing from it before it is safe. Cold expressed lime oil is phototoxic but a steam distilled one is not. There are several oils which have a question mark over their safety when used in other than trace amounts. Any natural oil, precisely because it is so concentrated, needs to be handled with care.

One of the main characteristics of low quality fragrances is the use of cheap fixatives. Natural perfumers have a plethora of high quality, very effective safe fixatives at their disposal. Likewise with the oils that contribute the middle notes which make up the body of any blend. When we get to the top notes it is more difficult for three reasons. Firstly, there are fewer natural top notes to choose from; secondly, their tenacity is low and finally, some are restricted. It is true that oils from the other categories are likewise restricted but because there are so many more to choose from, it is not such a blow. Bois de rose (rosewood) should not be used for environmental reasons (Guenther towards the end of the 19th Century warned about de-forestation and over exploitation). There are supposed to be tight controls in South America but much finds its way into the United States. Bitter Orange and nutmeg should only be used in small amounts. The question is, if one could enhance the quality and performance of an entirely natural product by the addition of small amounts of safe chemicals, should one do so? Would we have synthetics added to woollen socks to make them more hardwearing?

Whilst it is true that the cheapest so-called perfumes contain very cheap aldehydes, there are also some that are more costly and subtle. First used at the end of the nineteenth century, these synthetics were not initially seen as a substitute for natural oils but something which could add some radiance, lift and staying power to a natural blend. *Chanel No 5* was one of the first aldehyde perfumes to become famous. *Shalimar* was born by adding synthetic vanillin to an earlier Guerlain fragrance called *Jicky*. Edmound Roudnitska beautifully crafted *Diorissimo* after being commissioned by Christian Dior in 1957. Though based on Muguet (Lilly of the Valley, which is synthetic) it is much more than a single flower fragrance. It achieves what all good perfumes should: namely, a beautiful, homogenous scent that feels complete and rounded rather than an obvious blend of disparate elements that seem to lack harmony.

As children we used to talk about how the things we had never eaten tasted. The clue was, of course, in the smell which turns out to be very close to the adult reality of how we taste. As adults, there are smells that everybody knows despite never having smelled them. The example that comes to mind is that of the whore's handbag. So musk grains smell of sex. Incidentally, so does the Malacca Strait after spending ten days crossing the Indian Ocean by ship. Oh, and civet smells of shit.

There is a chemical called indole, which is found in absolutes derived from several white flowers including jasmine. It is also found in human faeces. Many repugnant odours, when sufficiently diluted, become pleasant and it is this principle that was utilised when using animal fixatives. It is also pertinent to consider how one's perception of odour changes during sexual arousal. So, why not try and create something so vile that not even Goths would wear it? I did and I dare you. The next step would be to create a homeopathic dose of the aforementioned that was so dilute that only a giant Barbie with fairy wings woven out of moth mohair could smell it. Okay, that's going too far but I do have a 100% botanical musk fixative.

In Ottoman cooking the cultivation of taste is preferred to following recipes. When one encounters a great wine something transcendent is present that can be recognised but never described. Hugh Johnson calls the process of creating such wines art. Our art should be about cultivation of aesthetic so that we can create in the service of beauty. How else can we know whether or not it is present?

FIVE

Cultivation, Taste and Consultations

At the end of the last chapter, I mentioned in relation to Ottoman cooking the tradition of preferring cultivation of taste to following written recipes. Likewise, in their traditional music, transmission was made aurally, rather than through trying to write the music down. In Western musical traditions there has been debate around the lack of musical indications given by Bach on many of his pieces. Some have argued that Bach assumed musicians capable of playing his pieces with their contrapuntal ingenuity and phrasing would instinctively know how to proceed correctly. Others prefer the view that Bach afforded considerable latitude to musicians to render their own interpretations. If one learns to taste wine professionally, what matters is being able to assess the quality of a wine, irrespective of whether or not one likes it. In professional wine examinations there is the expectation of being able to place a particular wine in hierarchical relation to others of similar type. One is also expected to be able to offer informed judgements on its age, where it is in terms of evolution, whether it will improve, if so, for how long and its current market value. Ultimately, consciously smelling a wine or a fragrance is a way of being very intimate with oneself. It is a very private matter and therefore totally subjective. However, in order to share and compare impressions a shared vocabulary is needed and that can only ever approximate. The reason is simple; despite the fact that each of us is equipped with a super sensitive olfactory bulb capable of distinguishing between 10,000 aromas, it seems that each of us is more sensitive to certain aromas than others. Further, we each have blind spots in certain parts of the aroma spectrum and to complicate matters further, can refer to the same aroma by different names. So how do we square this with objective assessment?

The American lawyer turned wine critic, Robert Parker, took it upon himself to score wines out of a possible 100. To some, this is the triumph of empiricism and to others, over simplistic reductionism. Can you imagine trying to score music out of 100? Personally, I have no doubt about Parker's integrity, but his influence has been far reaching and perhaps not always for the best. One New York wine merchant was reputed to say that he was unable to sell wines that Parker had scored under 90 and was unable to buy wines that Parker had scored over 90. Parker is known to favour heavily extracted wines that are usually quite intense and high in alcohol. Many winemakers have adjusted their winemaking techniques in order to produce wines that please such a palate, thereby ensuring higher scores, which mean higher prices. There are grapes, Pinot noir for example, that are incapable of producing such wines and retaining their identity, as their natural domain is more akin to finesse and delicacy.

It remains to be seen what long term effect the recently published *Perfumes The Guide* will have on fragrance fashion. In wine circles, at least on this side of the pond, it is commonly believed that US consumers are much happier to be told what to enjoy by the critics than consumers in Europe. The European notion that wine should have an identity that reminds one from where it comes is often dismissed as French greed posing as mysticism by many Americans. Why not just score'em? Our relationship with the American dream is still different from that of our buddies in the US but mind the gap. Do critics know best and how do we separate naked, raw and immediate experience from belief?

Brain scanning is able to help shed some light on extrinsic factors affecting assessment of aroma and wine. There is a relatively new technique called *f*MRI, or functional magnetic resonance imaging, that needs no radioactive materials and produces images at a high resolution. It is based on differences in the magnetic resonance of certain atomic nuclei in areas of neuronal activity, making it possible to observe in subjects which parts of their brains are most active. Discrete areas of the brain are responsible for diverse activities. In one experiment participants were given wines and were told that the wines cost $5, $10, $35, $45 or $90 respectively and were asked to comment on how pleasurable each was. Despite the real cost, participants rated the wines labelled with higher prices as being more pleasurable. Interestingly, the *f*MRI data appeared to show real increased pleasure despite all the wines being identical. The scanner was able to monitor changes in the medial orbito-frontal cortex, which is associated with an increase of pleasure (quoted by Thomas, 2008, p.380).

It may seem obvious to state that the colour of a wine influences our assessment, but just how much is surprising. Some tastings now use black glasses in an attempt to minimise such effects. Thomas refers to another experiment (Osterbauer et al. 2005), which involved adding odourless, red dye to white wine. This fooled even Masters of wine into describing the 'nose' in terms usually reserved for describing red wines. These effects were shown to modify the response to an aroma directly in the primary olfactory cortex. So a Day-Glo orange wine would not only look bizarre, but would also smell peculiar. Other experiments showed that verbalising scent impressions completely undermined the performance in novice tasters being asked to taste wines, and later match them with others from a large selection. Novices diminished their success by attempting to describe the wines between tasting the first set of wines and attempting to match them with wines from the second group. However, when they did not verbalise their impressions between tasting and selection, their performance matched that of experts. It was also found that experts were able to discriminate between, and match, sets of wines that novices found indistinguishable. A further experiment, again quoted by Thomas (Castriota-Scanderberg and colleagues 2005), demonstrated that sommeliers brain activity when tasting was different from that of novice control subjects. The difference was attributed to a learned ability to integrate sensory information from taste and smell with past experience. In addition, the sommeliers showed activation in parts of the brain associated with high level cognitive processes such as working memory and behavioural strategies. The difference between the sommeliers and the novices was not so much in their ability to detect aromas but the fact that the novices just lacked the knowledge and memory of similar experience available to the sommeliers.

These findings have confirmed what many have known through experience and commonsense. After learning to taste wine, it is usual to proceed with the study of individual grape varieties in relation to different geographical areas of cultivation and winemaking styles. Colour and other visual clues are so important. Merlot will never have the deep purple of a ripe young Cabernet Sauvignon and Pinot Noir, however ripe, will never be black like Syrah. Imagine having filed in the brain a microfiche containing all the information that one has learned in relation to a particular grape variety or winemaking region. The visual clues offered by inspecting a glass of wine prompt a search for the most relevant microfiche. The information on this microfiche then becomes a kind of mental lens through which one experiences the wine. It is similar to the process of tuning an old-fashioned wireless set with a dial. For example, if I see a glass of almost water white wine with a slight greenish hue, the microfiches for Riesling, Sauvignon Blanc, Albarino and Fino Sherry will be on standby. A quick sniff rules out the almond, yeastiness of the Fino. So the microfiche is instantly returned to the library. Inhaling more deeply, a very delicate light elderflower quality reveals itself. The Albarino microfiche is also returned to the library. I also notice underneath the delicate floral characteristics hints of beeswax and honey. The Sauvignon is too light in colour to have sufficient ripeness to exhibit these characteristics so that microfiche, too, is filed. On my Riesling microfiche is a range of possibilities that start with elderflower and progress through linden blossom, beeswax, lemon, lime, grapefruit, green apples, stony minerals, paint thinners, wet wool, petrol and diesel. Attached to each one of these aromas is another file containing information about soil types, weather patterns, microclimates, effects of bottle ageing, Riesling producing areas, and all my personal experiences of Riesling. I now use my awareness, combined with the sense of smell to tune in as specifically as I can to the aroma characteristics of the wine. As I taste the wine, my curiosity will be looking to see if the tasting impressions support or negate any of the information supplied by my nose. In the mouth it is light, not at all oily, has marked citrus acidity, very delicate flavours suggestive of minerals, exhibits a slight honey-like sweetness, is low in alcohol, nicely balanced and has a very long finish. For such a wine, my experience would suggest a young Spätlese from a top producer in the Moselle region of Germany.

In support of the 'duped' Masters of wine I would like to suggest that instant de- coupling from mental pathways that have taken decades to cultivate may not be possible. Remember the sommeliers, whose capacity was a product of the relationship between sensory information and memory. It is also possible that as our sense of smell is so sensitive and the range of recognisable aromas so vast that characteristics normally associated with red wines were discernible to highly trained noses in the dyed white wines. I remember some years ago being invited to a vertical tasting of Lopez de Heredia's Vina Tondonia, one of the only bodegas that is still making traditional Rioja. When confronted by the 1964 white Rioja, one of the tasters suggested how easily it could be mistaken for a red Rioja if tasted blind. Several people rolled their eyes in mocking disbelief. The response from the winemaker was nice and clear: 'That is what my grandfather says.'

So, what does all this have to do with perfume? The salient points are that novices can smell as well as experts, and that engaging the rational part of brain may support the expert, but is unhelpful to the novice. The knowledge available to the expert comprises factual information and a memory bank of relevant experience. Different parts of the brain are involved in detecting aromas and assessing them. For the novice, who lacks a working connection between these two capacities, their awareness can perhaps only focus on one or the other but not both simultaneously. We know that smell, like music, goes straight to the part of the brain that stimulates emotions rather than the part that controls our speech. This means that we can have an instinctual response to an aroma, but find it hard to verbalise. It also means that our verbosity can interfere with the instinctual response.

According to one prevalent theory, the brain has evolved into a triune structure that has been described as a crocodile, a horse and a person. The oldest part of the brain, the so called 'R complex', is reptilian and is only interested in survival and procreation. The next part, called the 'limbic system', is mammalian and capable of much more complex social interaction than a crocodile. Finally, along came the new kid on the block called the 'neocortex', or Mister clever clogs, the rational part, which is perhaps only 40,000 years old.

A crocodile doesn't worry about eating a baby gnu in front of mummy gnu. Neither, as far as we know, does it compare the tenderness of today's gnu with the one it ate last Thursday. When living in Bristol, I used to visit the zoo quite frequently and got to know some of the keepers and animals. The keepers get to know the animals intimately and can tell immediately if the giraffe or the red panda is having a bad hair day. Reptiles are different – there is absolutely no indication or way of knowing just what is going on inside. Their range of social activity is quite restricted in relation to mammals.

We have some neighbours who've been feeding badgers regularly for some years. The badgers have become quite tame, and some will even take food from the hand. A young badger has learnt that if he ignores the food on the ground and begs by the house his behaviour is rewarded by tastier morsels. For a while, the family of badgers even adopted two orphaned fox cubs, who would accompany them for their evening meal. Badgers, being nocturnal, feed at night and by sunrise are usually well snuffled underground. On one occasion, our neighbours woke to find two badgers waiting by the house. One badger was badly injured; the other, its companion, was healthy. The injured badger was taken to the vet, who was able to help before it was reunited with its friends.

The rational part of the brain is concerned with language, planning and ideas.

When I am asked to make a unique fragrance for a client the starting point is a consultation. During the consultation process I try and discover the client's instinctual response to each of a group of 60 completely natural, single note fragrances. At this point in the consultation, the contents of each bottle are not disclosed to the client. Each bottle is offered in turn, and the client is invited to respond to each aroma with a simple yes or no. Any further embellishment would usually take the client away from the immediacy of their instinctual response. For the process to work well we must try to catch the immediate, instinctual response to each fragrance. The instinctual response is a subtle, energetic movement either towards or away from the contents of the bottle. Attraction or repulsion only, rationality is not involved other than in sharing the response. The 60 fragrances are gone through in a certain order, to avoid stronger aromas masking more delicate ones. All the 'yes' bottles are left on the table, and the 'no' bottles returned to the box.

At this point, we can now start discussing contents of each bottle. Usually, themes emerge. Some clients, for example, may not be drawn to citrus or floral aromas but like balsams instead. During each consultation it is really important that I do not influence clients at all. As we have seen from the wines with the most expensive labels, it would be quite easy to get a client to select nearly any bottle I chose. Most of the oils and absolutes have a long and interesting history. Many have romantic stories from folklore and others, tales of how rare and precious they are. By involving the imagination, the emperor's new clothes effect can seduce clients away from their instinctual response.

There is a third experiential place where one is just in the experience of smelling the aroma without any judgement of like or dislike. It is useful to be able to experience aromas in this way, as it helps one to 'learn' them by imprinting them on the nervous system. Clients sometimes find themselves in this state when they have a neutral response to one of the fragrances, in which case, I leave it as a 'maybe' and we return to it later. During consultations, I will always smell each bottle before passing it to the client as a way of reinforcing my familiarity with each.

The number of 'yes' bottles on the table can vary enormously between clients. My task now is to sort the 'yes' bottles into groups and decide with the client what the structure of their unique fragrance will be. At this point, I'm more than happy to share information about each fragrance with the client and the consultation process becomes much more convivial. Rather than talk about the fragrance in terms of top, middle and base notes, I have evolved some other terminology, which clients find easier to relate to. It also helps me to envisage possible fragrance structures. I use the terms *heart, nuance and intrigue.*® The heart will be the main body of the fragrance, imagine it at the centre of a circle. It could be simple and based upon a single flower or complex, involving many accords. Around the heart we build nuance, using compatible fragrances, which add depth, subtlety and colour. Assuming a floral heart, we may use wood, citrus or a blend of both to impart nuances. The outer circle belongs to intrigue, whose job it is to invite curiosity, originality and interest.

The interesting thing about blending, and this is particularly true about intrigue, is that oils and absolutes can be included well below the threshold of conscious detection, but they still have a major impact on the final fragrance. Once I have decided with the client upon the structure of their fragrance based upon this model of *heart, nuance and intrigue,*® the consultation is over.

The next part of the process involves me making up two samples which are sent to the client through the post. I encourage each client to wear both simultaneously, one on each wrist, and to constantly smell them during the day, to reapply them at bedtime and see how they are in the morning. Friends and lovers should be involved. In this way, the client gets to know each and how they interact with the person's own smell and metabolism. After a few days a telephone conversation with the client takes place in order to get feedback. Most usually the client will choose one or the other; occasionally they require more time to make their choice, or will simply have both. It is also possible to give a final 'tweak' to one of the samples to make it more floral, woody, spicy, herby, musky etc. before sending the finished fragrance.

A French perfumer called Jean Charles outlined in some detail a systematic way of creating fragrances based upon the blending of accords. An accord is a blend of two or more notes. If one is interested in learning to blend fragrances and have access to aromatic raw materials it is a very effective learning tool. Not only does it increase familiarity with the aromatic raw materials, but also, more importantly, the interaction between them. I shall outline the basic method as it can demonstrate something interesting about taste and subjectivity as a useful conclusion to this chapter.

Supposing we need to create an Oriental style perfume, and we decide to start working from the bottom up. Initially, we choose patchouli, vetivert and labdanum to form a basic accord. The method of Jean Charles is going to be used to decide upon the precise proportion of each of the oils in this blend. We proceed by making up blends in the following proportions.

Patchouli	9	8	7	6	5
Vetivert	1	2	3	4	5

After mixing each blend thoroughly we can evaluate them using smelling strips. We select the one that we consider to be the most appropriate and also decide to incorporate labdanum. Let's assume that the most suitable for our purposes is that with the ratio of 7:3 of patchouli to vetivert. We may repeat the exercise as follows:-

7:3 Patchouli:					
Vetivert blend	9	8	7	6	5
Labdanum	1	2	3	4	5

After mixing each of the new blends thoroughly, we again use smelling strips to evaluate them. After careful consideration, we select the one most suitable for our purposes and we decide that it is the one with the ratio of 8:2 patchouli: vetivert blend to labdanum. We could carry on in this manner, constructing a more complex base by incorporating clary sage absolute, beeswax absolute, opopanax, frankincense and lashings of sandalwood. Once we are happy with our base we may wish to introduce some floral accords to modify it. Now we have a choice: we can either blend our floral accord before incorporating it within the base or we simply begin adding floral notes, one at a time, to the base. Being oriental, jasmine suggests itself immediately; we may wish to warm it with a hint of caraway and soften it with rose maroc before imparting lift with neroli. It is important to realise that we can act outside of these ratios. Some of the spice oils need handling with extreme caution to prevent them from losing their usefulness. If we are assessing an accord in the ratios of 9:1 it is quite possible that for some oils that 1 will be much too high a concentration. In which case, if we want to persist with it, we may drop down to 0.5, or even 0.1.

In relation to both wine tasting and fragrance blending, I cannot emphasise strongly enough the value of working in a group. Quite apart from the fact that it's much more fun than trying to be a solitary genius, some people's receptors are capable of detecting extraordinary nuances. When these perceptions are shared, it enables everyone in the group to focus their enquiry into areas that they may never have stumbled across on their own.

In conclusion, I would like to say that when working with ratios in a group I am always astonished during assessment by the quorum consensus. So maybe those old Ottoman cooks were correct in insisting that taste could be cultivated and such an individual would instinctively know when things were right.

▶ *The painting describes the history of natural perfume using images and symbols, which depict significant plant materials, places and historical events. The central panel depicts the energy of polarity and procreation which 'drives' the historical process. The first part of chapter one alludes to the main historical and cultural factors portrayed. Elsewhere in the book you will find clues about the significance of other images in the work. Limited edition prints on archival paper are available in hand made mounts and frames using traditional gesso techniques.*
(Print size 75cm x 75cm. Size including frame and mount 110cm x 110cm).

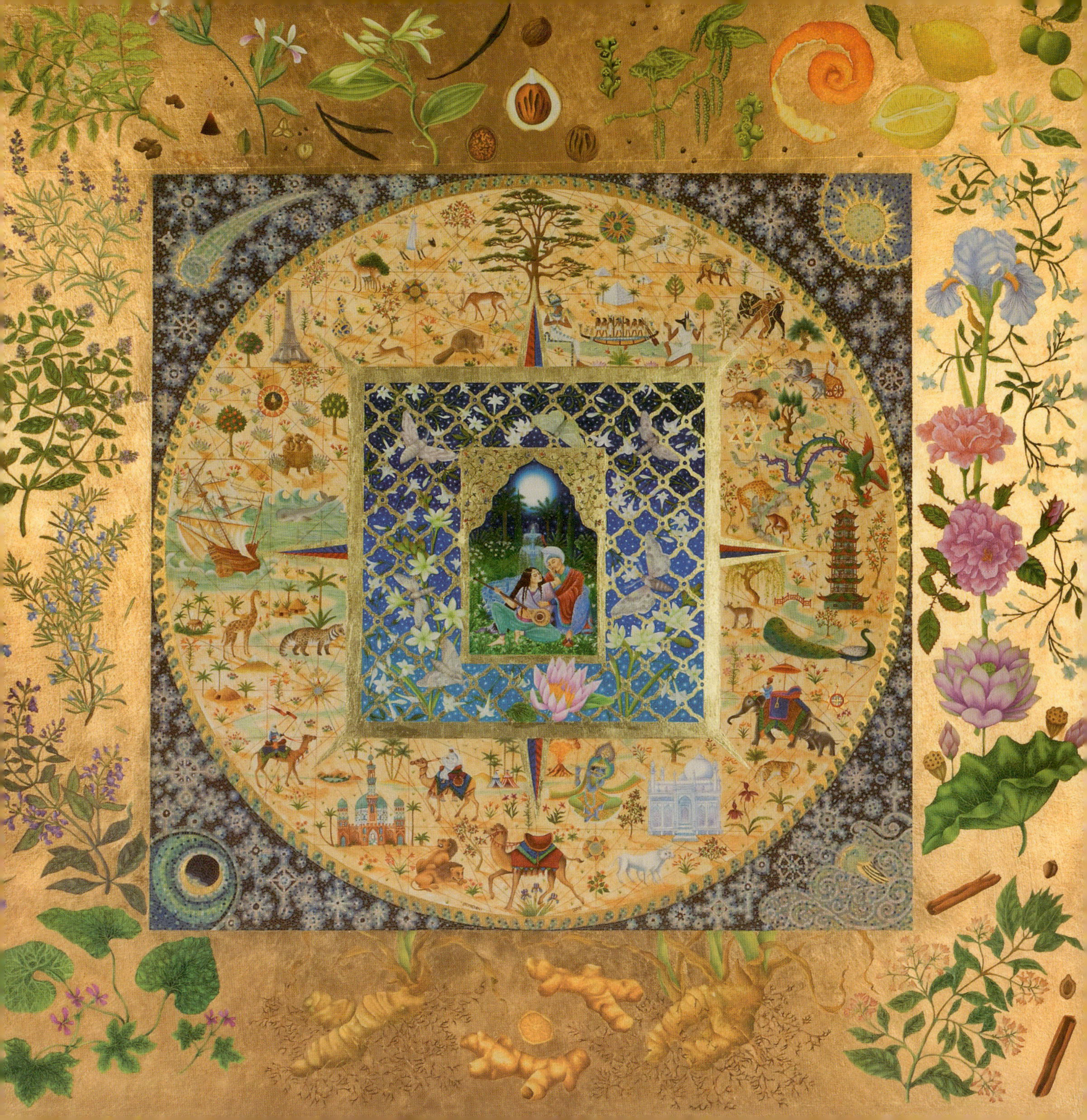

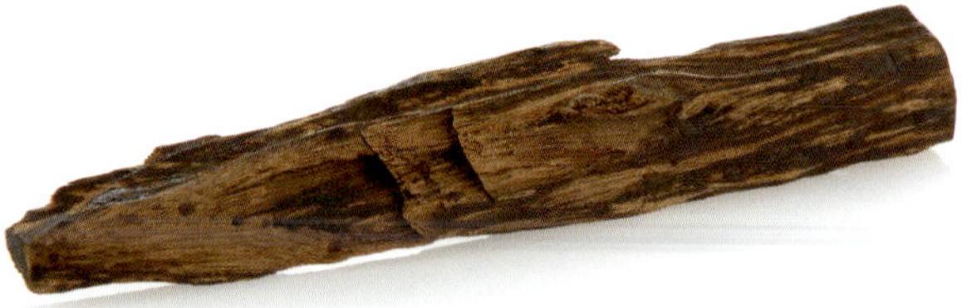

▲ **Aloewood** *Also known by many other names including agar wood. Originally from China, the oil formed the basis of the legendary Arabian perfume called Owd, Oud or Aud. It came to Europe during the 8th Century AD. See introduction for more information about aloewood.*

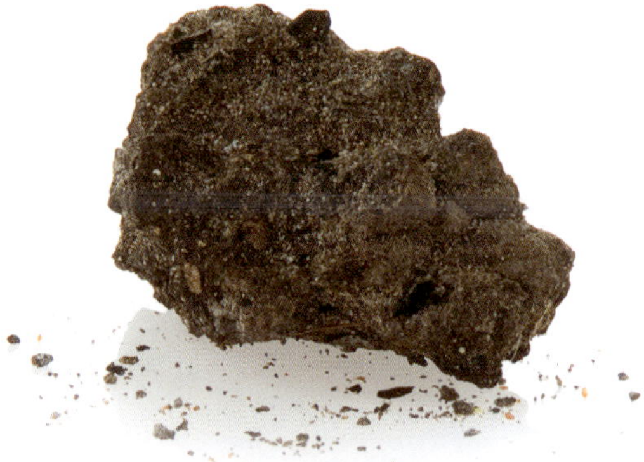

▲ **Ambergris** *One of the most valuable substances in the ancient world.*

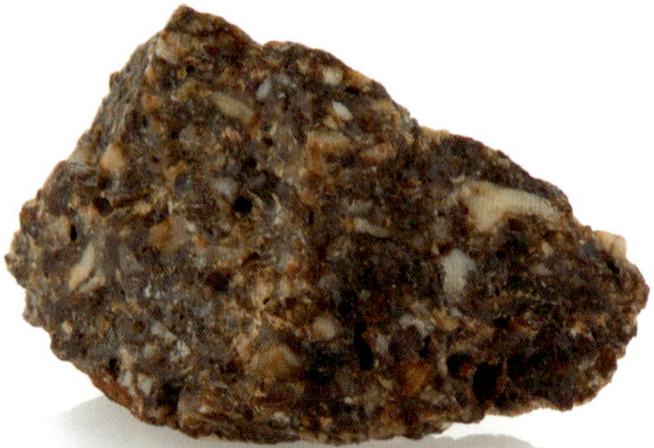

▲ **Crude Benzoin** *Crude benzoin or gum Benjamin as it was also known in the ancient world. This piece is solid like very hard toffee. The oil is very thick and viscous at room temperature so it needs a diluent to make it mobile.*

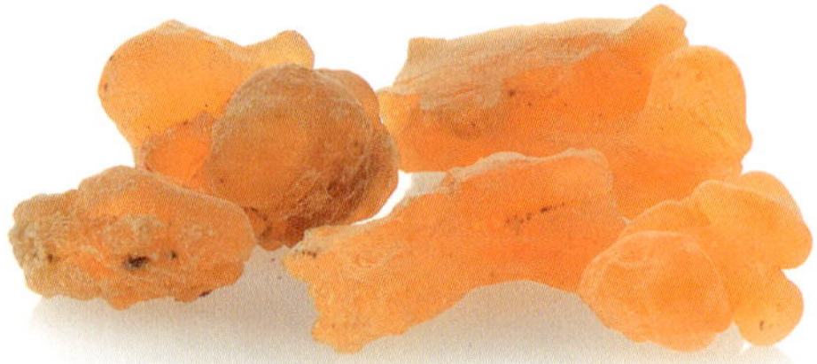

▲ **Frankincense Tears** *Frankincense resin is a pathological secretion from the small tree Boswellia carteri. The oleo gum resin becomes hard and brittle when exposed to oxygen. Frankincense tears were used as currency in the ancient world. The oil or absolute is extracted from the tears. Tears can also be burnt on charcoal and used as incense.*

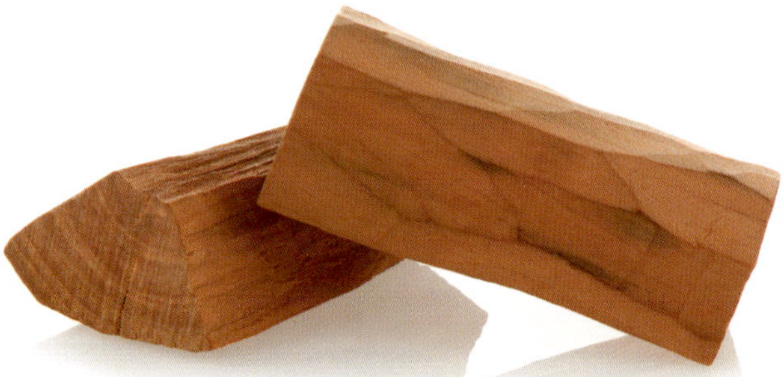

▲ **Mysore Sandalwood** *The best oil is extracted from the roots and the wood at the base of the tree.*

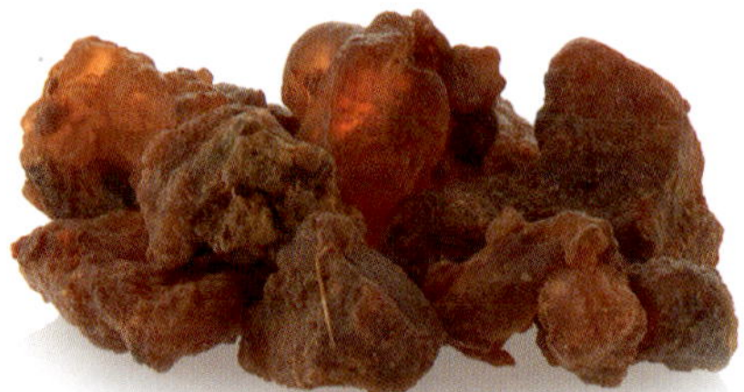

▲ **Myrrh Resin** *Bitter perfume and gathering gloom? We'll we like it more than that. Like frankincense, the resin is a pathological secretion from the tree Commiphora myrrha, which hardens when exposed to the oxygen. The oil or absolute is extracted from the hardened resin.*

Teddy delivering lavender from Provence.

The location of the field that produces this high altitude lavender is secret. I don't even know where it is. Harvest time is decided by a seer at Glastonbury who channels a dolphin who in a past life controlled lavender production on Atlantis. When I get the nod from her I go there to supervise the selection of perfect flowering heads. I am blindfolded and taken the last 20 km by Jean Le Brec. Peter Mayle picks the flowers one at a time and passes them to me for 'blind' selection. Only the most pristine examples that are considered 'à point' make it into Teddy's basket. The journey back by donkey enables the lavender to dry slowly as nature intended. Donkey delivered lavender has time to acclimatise gradually to changing humidity and temperature on its journey to the UK. The resultant oil is completely free from the mal odours associated with distillation of 'shocked' lavender delivered by post-industrialised mechanised means. The healing energy in the oil is so powerful that distribution is restricted to aromatherapists who have completed our most advanced training. In the wrong hands it could be dangerous. Teddy seems to know when he is carrying lavender and is seen here checking his load. Something he never does when carrying other cargo. The price is high for obvious reasons. Recently, lead times have increased considerably as we now avoid the Toulouse area and travel a more circuitous route. Teddy had some problems with a drunken chef wielding salami whilst passing through during the garlic festival.

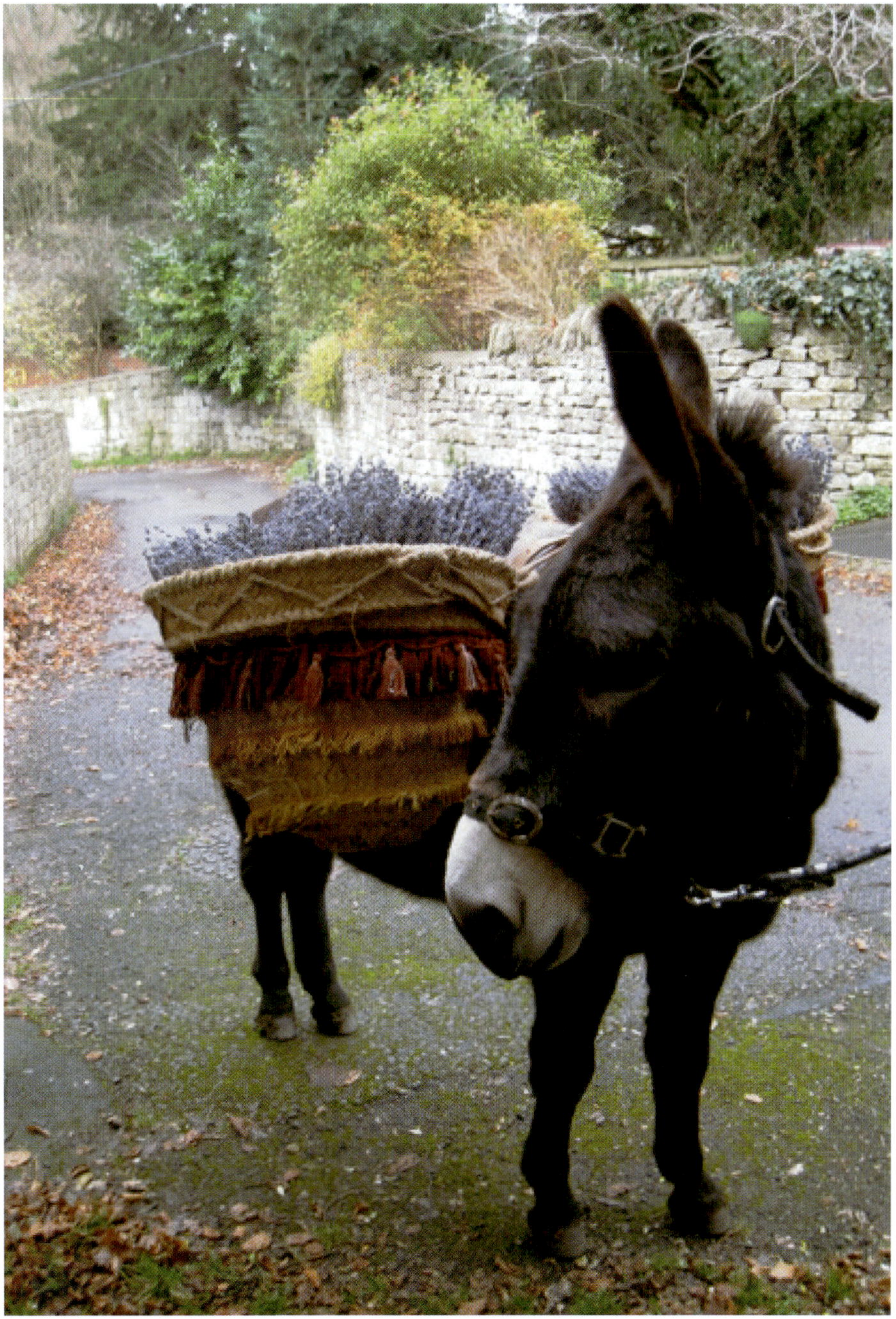

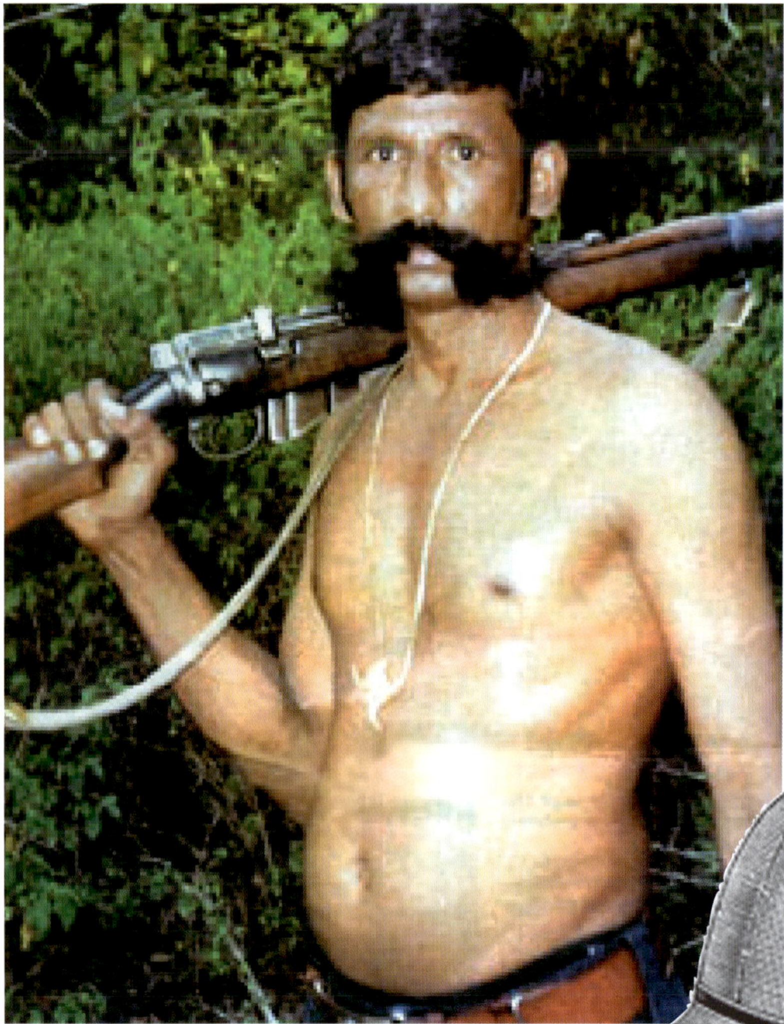

◄ **Koose Munisawamy Veerappan.**
Here he is with his gun. He was shot dead on October 18th 2004 after a tip off. The bounty on his head was 20 million rupees (about £250,000 at the time). Ten years earlier he had eluded a force of nearly 2,000 police officers who combed the forest looking for him. He is reported to have shot more than 120 forest official and over 2000 elephants during his lifetime. The survival of local tigers is now seriously under threat due to the insatiable demand from Chinese medicine.

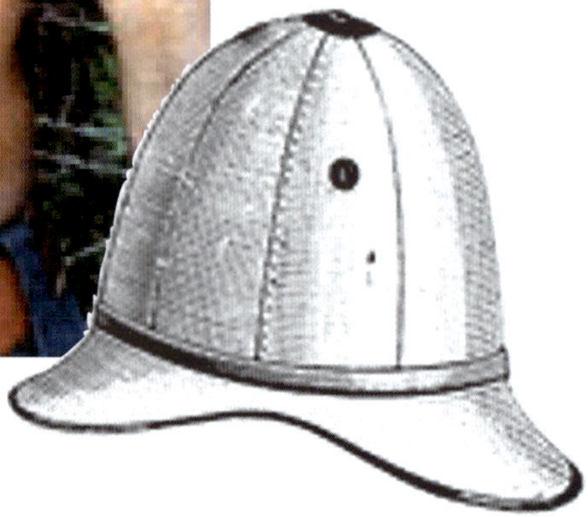

▲ **Colonial Topee.**
Originated in India to protect Colonials' fair skin from the sun. Named after the Hindi for hat. Usage later spread to Africa.

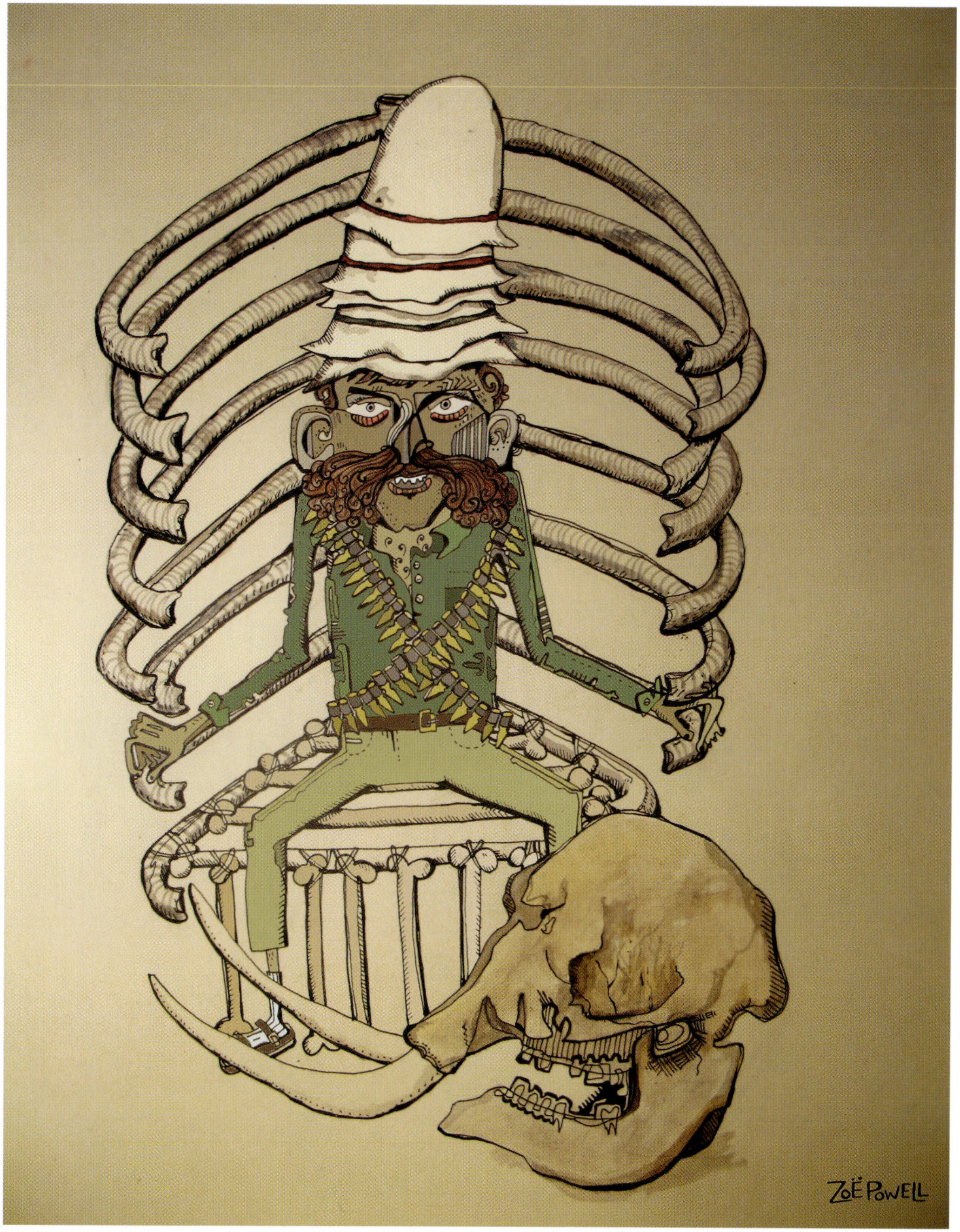

▶ **Veerappan's Topee**
As you can see, Sahib Veerappan beat the Colonials at their own game. Picture courtesy of Zoe P. Mysore Museum of Imaginal Anthropology.

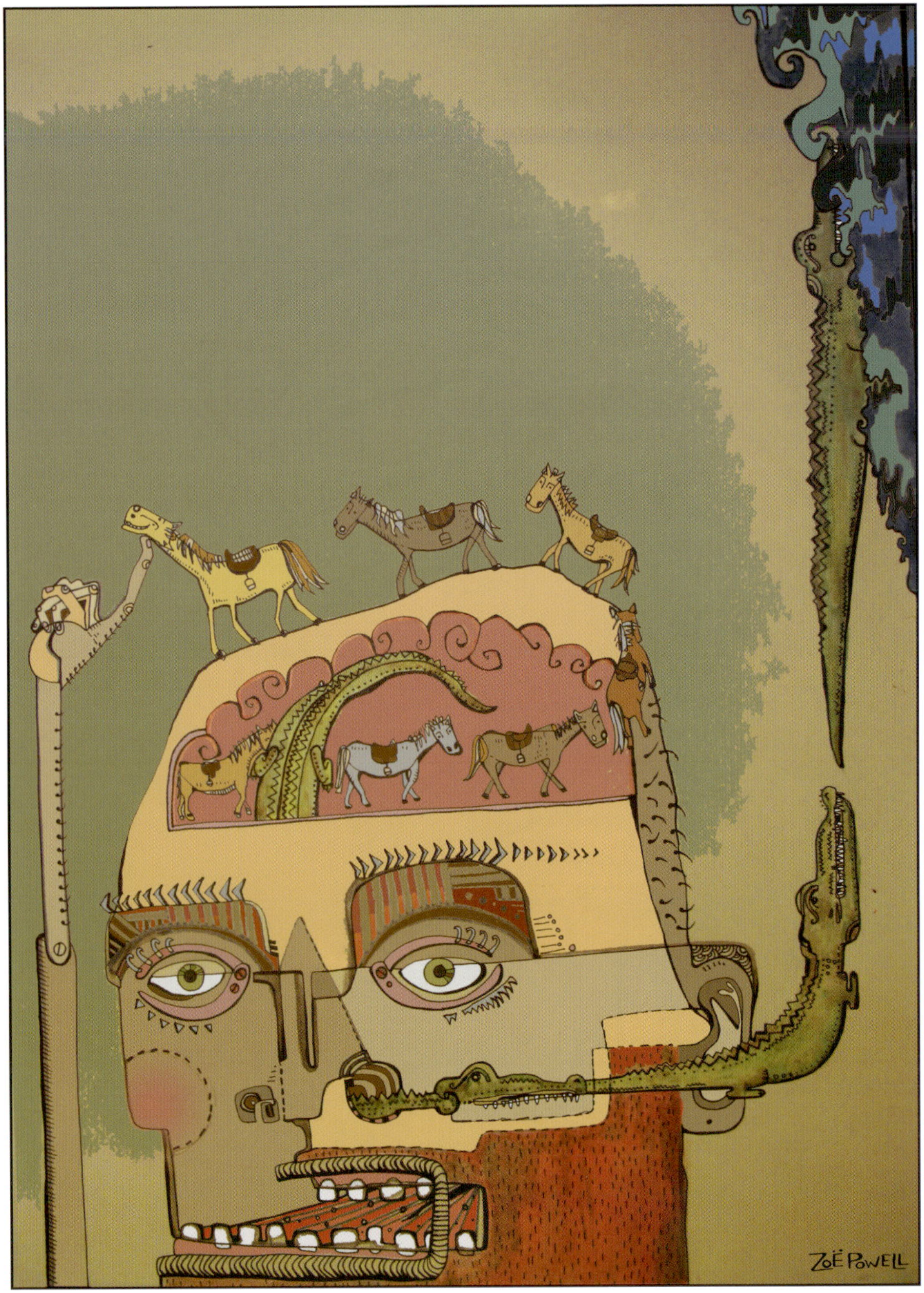

The Brain and Smell.
Courtesy of Zoe P. Institute of Experiential Brain Evolution Imaging.

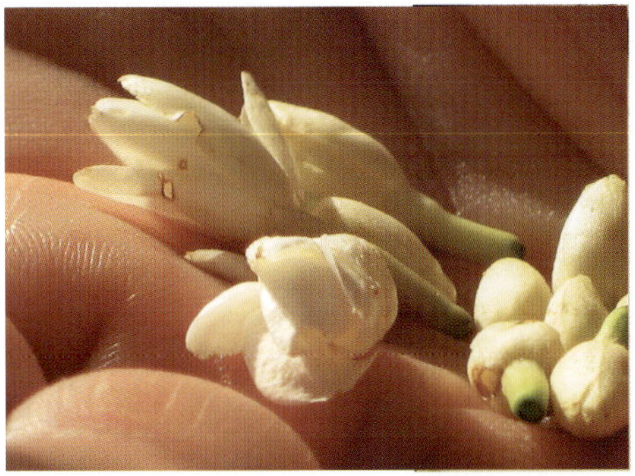

▲ *The author holding fresh champac flowers, India October 2008.*

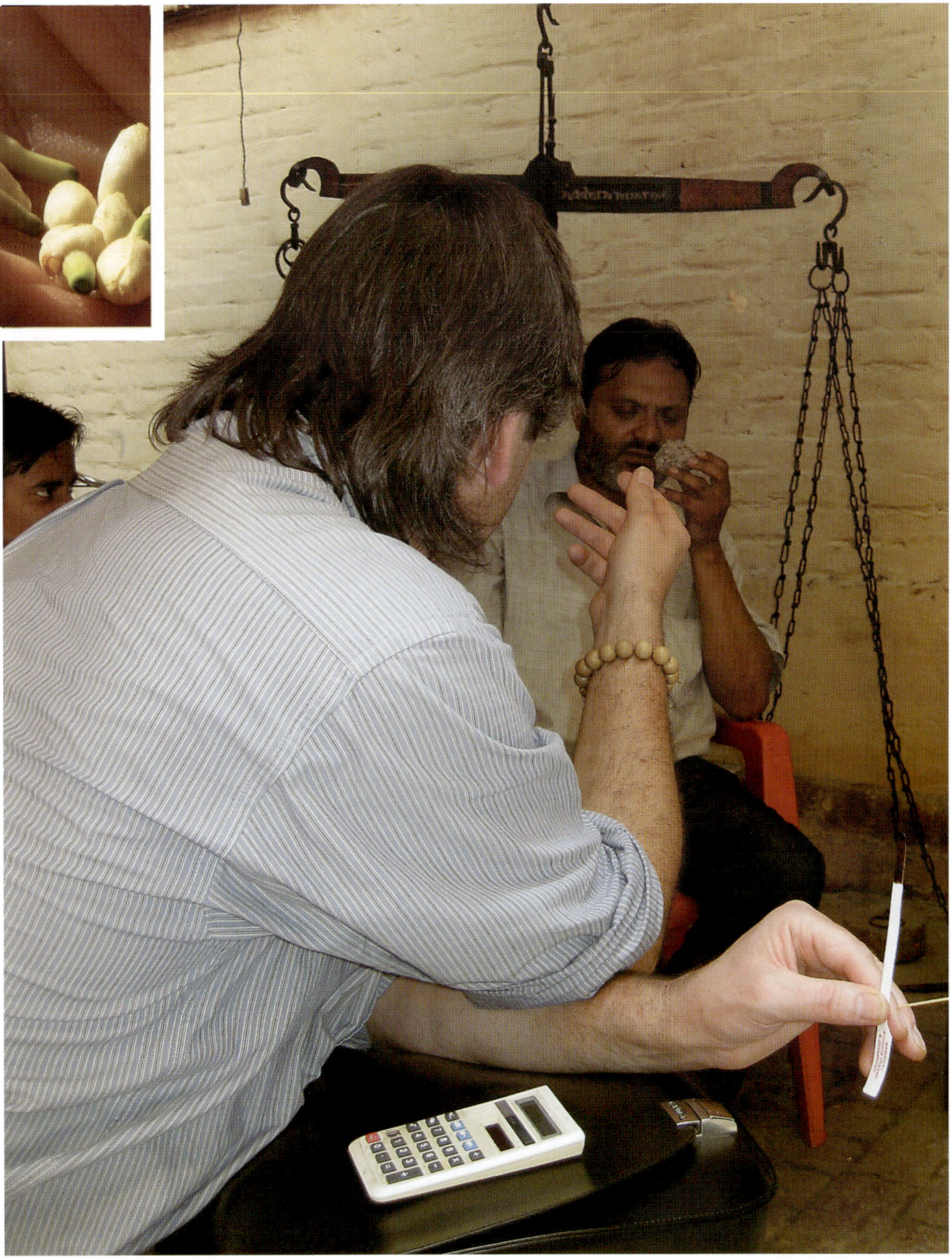

► *Author with friend and translator, Tanu, India October 2008.*

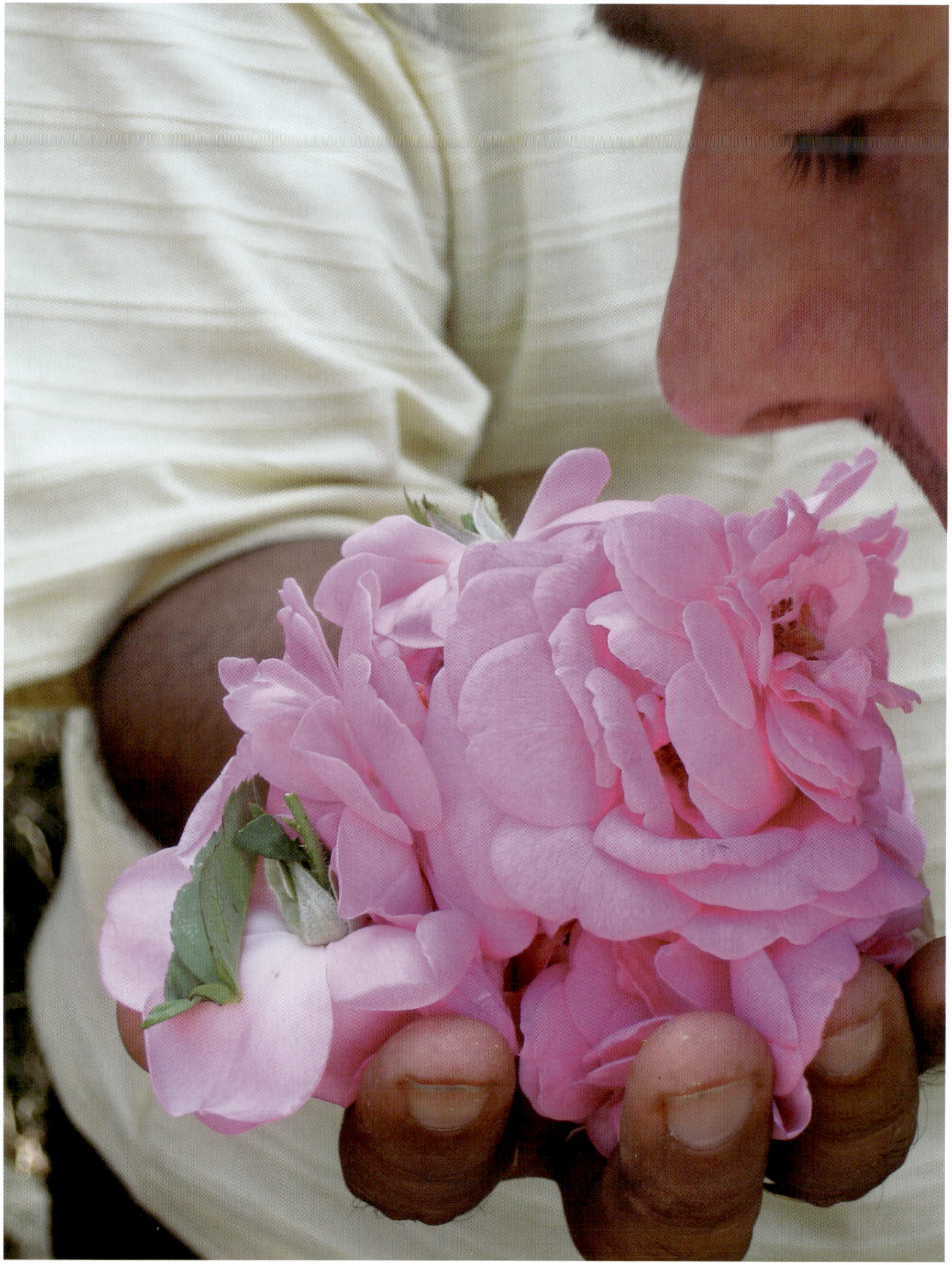

The author smelling the rose petals before they go into the still. India October 2008.

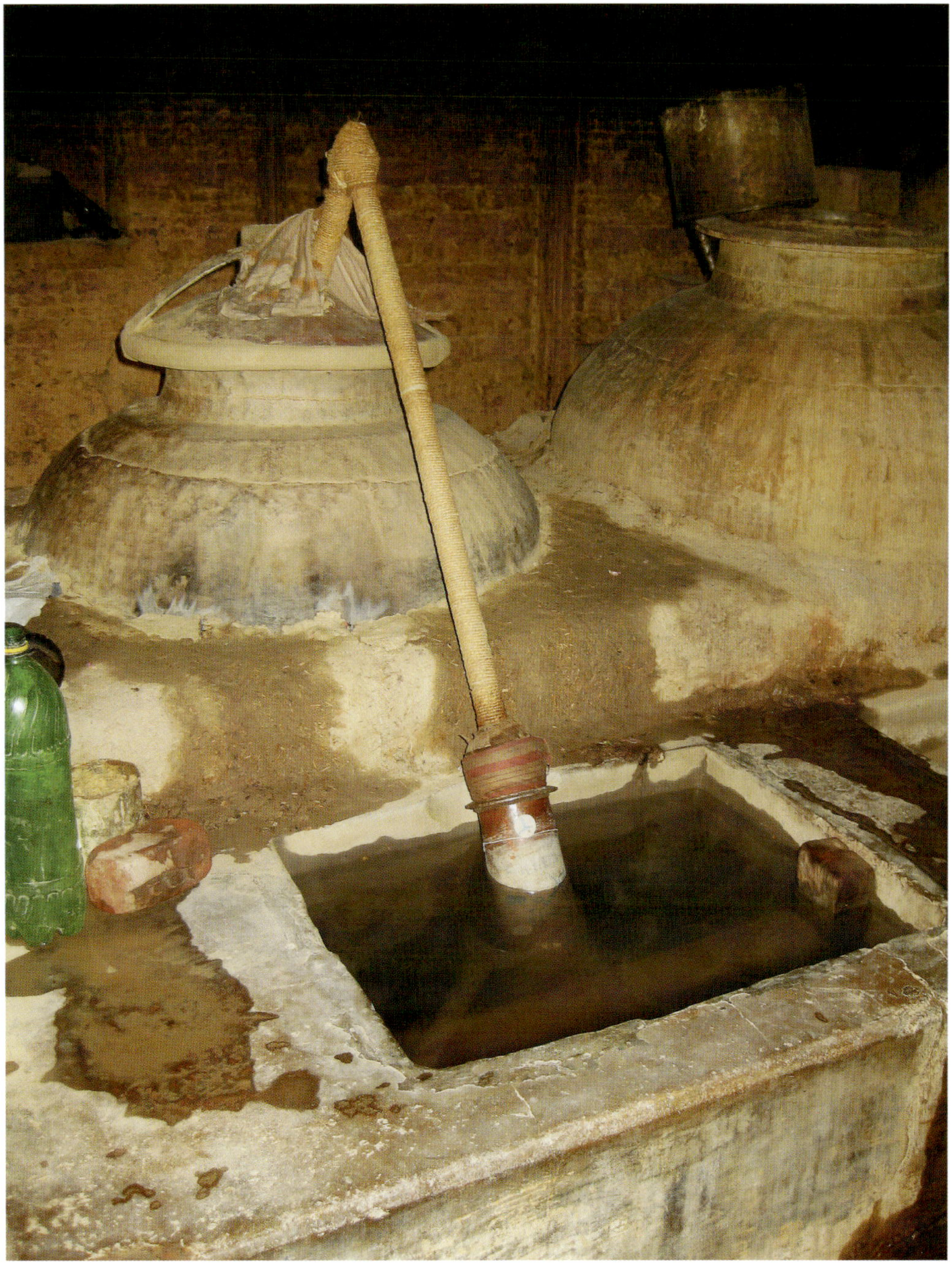

Hydro distillation has been practised in parts of India for centuries. The extracted essential oils were added to a base of sandalwood oil from Mysore and sold as traditional attars.

The copper still contains water and rose petals and is heated by a log fire to boil the water. The steam, along with rose oil that has evaporated, leaves the still under pressure and makes its way down the pipe into the container immersed in water. The cooling effect of the water forces the steam to condense. The resultant distillate is water with rose oil floating on top.

The rope is wrapped around the pipe to make it safe to touch. The cooling water needs changing frequently as it becomes quite warm after an hour or so. This process is continued over many days. India October 2008.

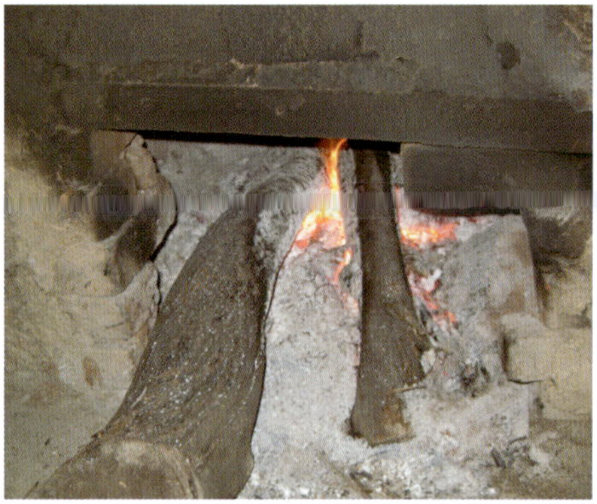

▲ *Logs under the still heating the water. India October 2008.*

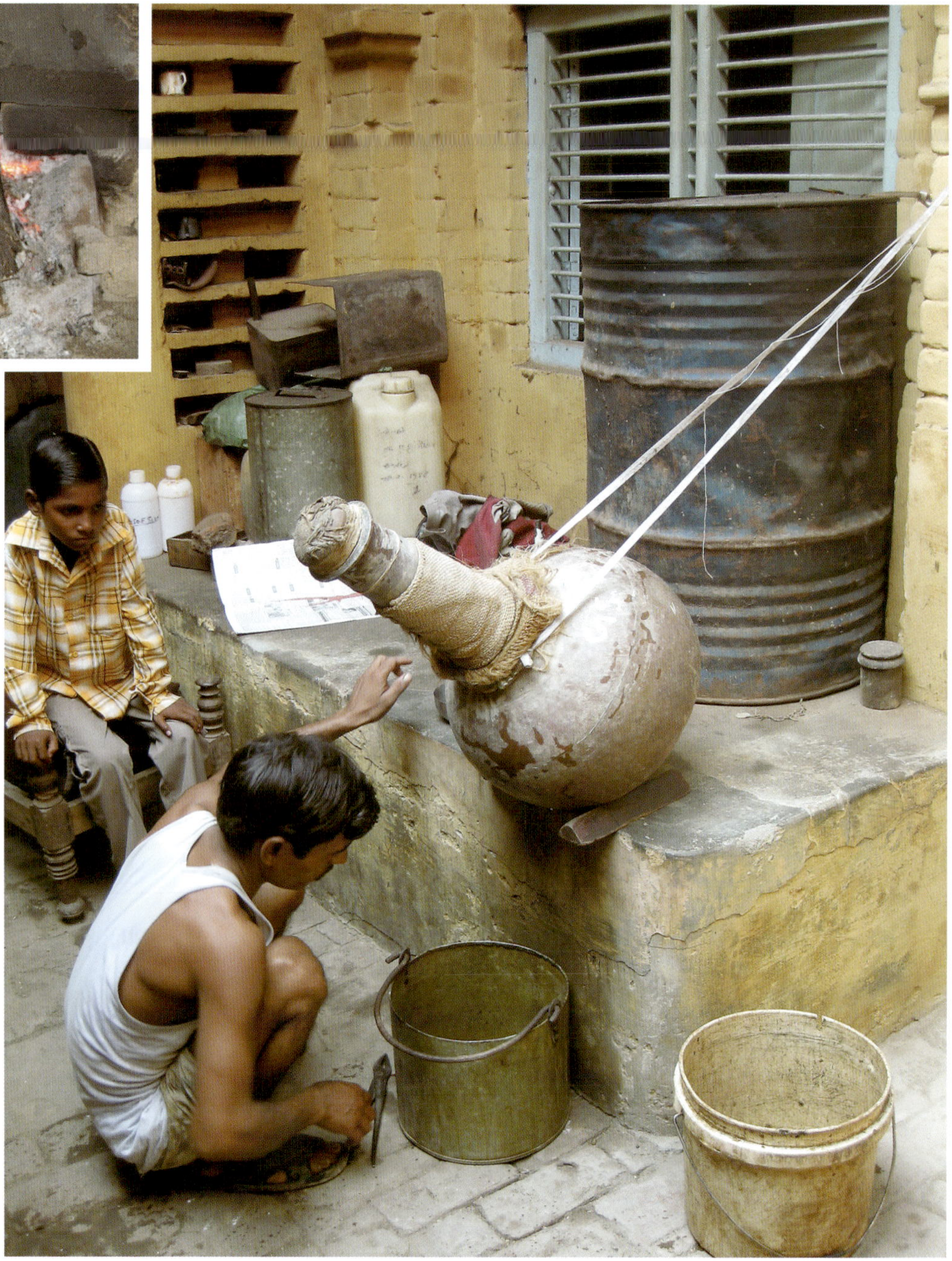

▶ *The condensation vessel has a bung in its side which is removed before carefully tilting the vessel and allowing the water to flow out of the hole into a container. The condensed oil is floating on the water so all the water will leave the vessel before any of the rose oil. The water is returned to the still and used over and over again with fresh batches of rose petals. India October 2008.*

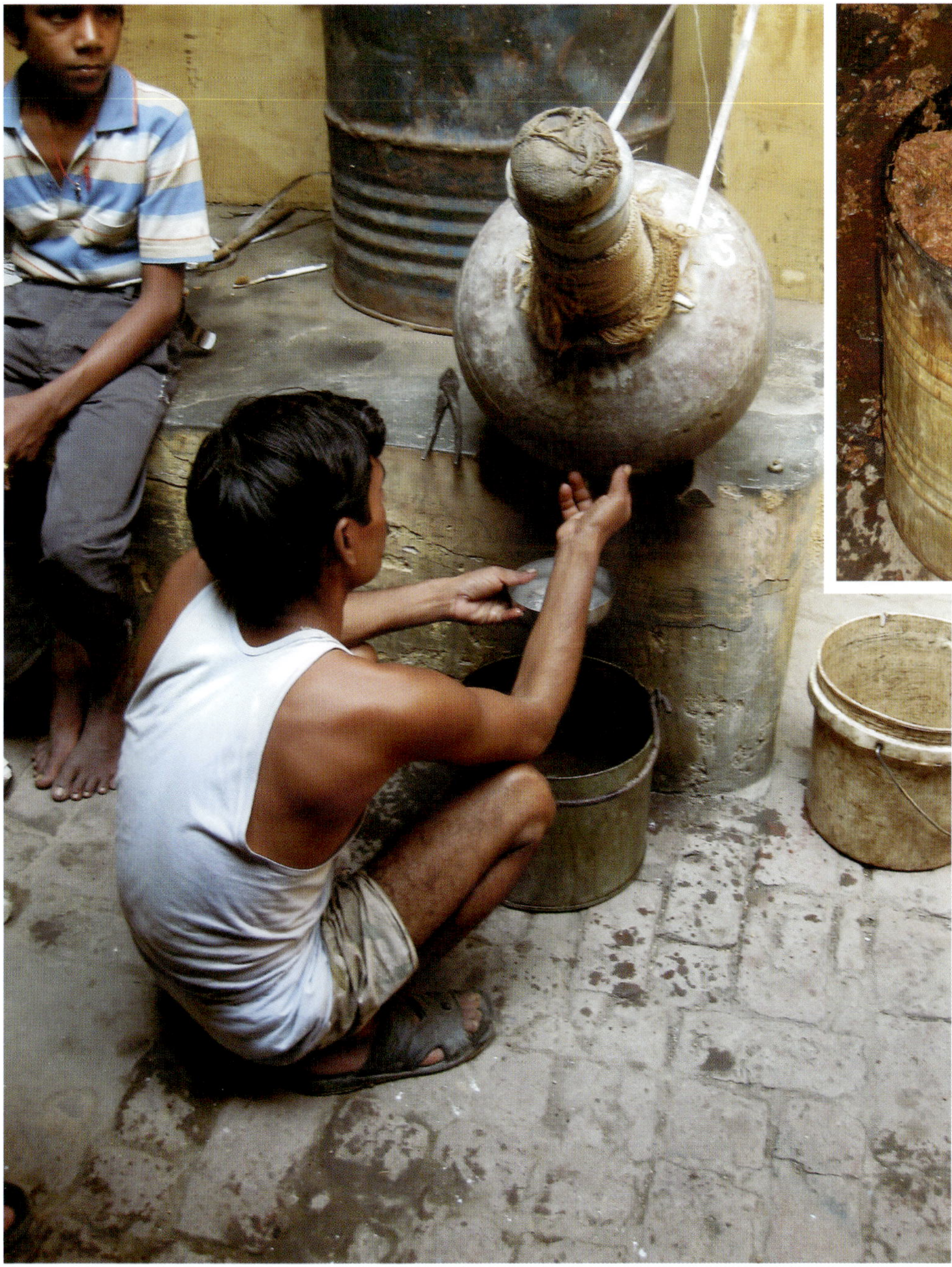

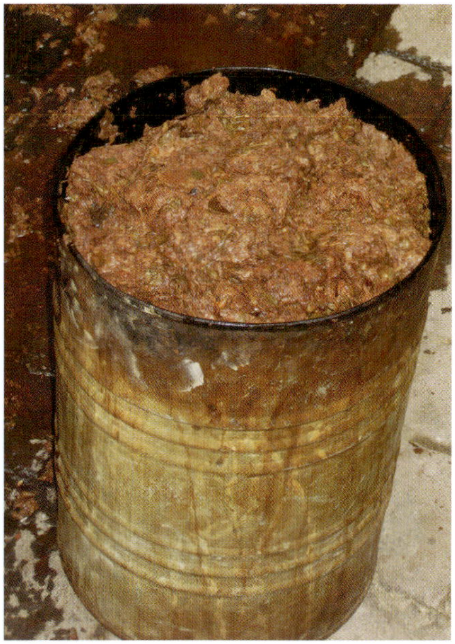

▲ *The rose petals after they have rendered their precious gift.*

◄ *The water is seen leaving the still and being caught in a bowl. As soon as any rose oil is seen, the flow is stopped by pressing a finger over the hole. The vessel is returned to an upright position when the bung can be safely replaced to preserve the precious contents. India October 2008.*

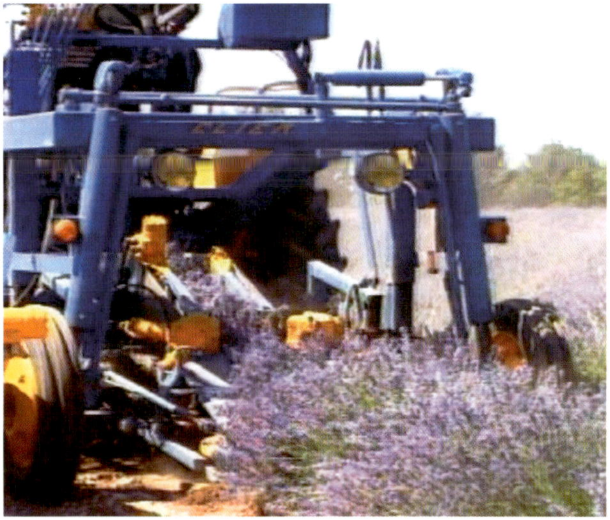

▲ *Lavender harvest, Southern France.*

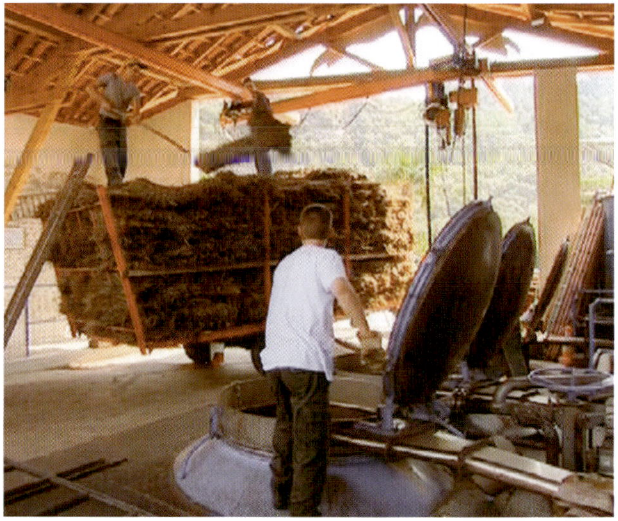

▲ *Loading the still with bundles of lavender, Southern France.*

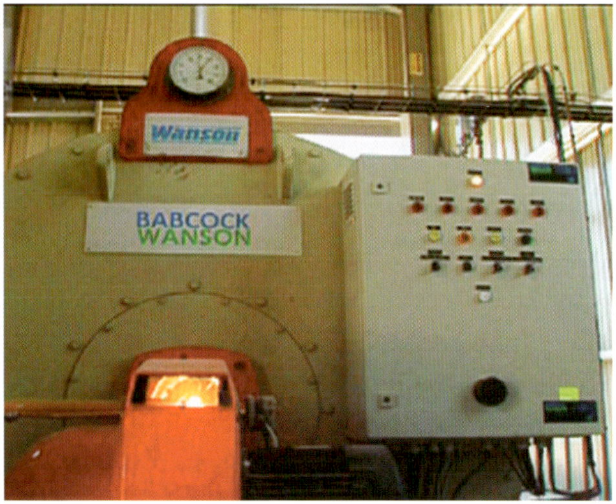

▲ *Modern gas furnace, Southern France.*

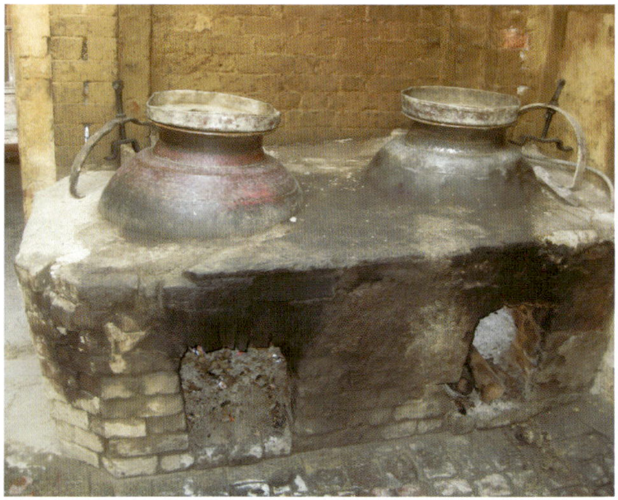

▲ *A pair of old stills, Central India.*

SIX

A Word about Blending

The great wine writer, Hugh Johnson, considers that scientific decisions are made on the basis of measurements, non-scientific decisions on the basis of habit, intuition or occasionally inspiration. Deciding where to draw the line between craftsmanship and art, he suggests that the first two are craftsmanship and only the third art. However, intuition or inspiration cannot happen in a vacuum. The inspiration behind Kekule's vision of the benzene ring, Beethoven's compositions after he went deaf, or Einstein's musings about relativity all took form within their specialist areas of knowledge. These inspired creative leaps, by definition, always go beyond the rules. However, could the pianist Joanna McGregor, who according to the Irish Times doesn't so much break down barriers but refuses to acknowledge that they exist, play like she does without years of disciplined classical study? It is true that occasionally a Jimi Hendrix comes along but for the rest of us we must do some donkeywork to prepare the ground in our given field of study.

Ultimately, there are no rules in perfumery but before we abandon ourselves in the dark to our muse, it is wise to become thoroughly familiar with the basics. These basics are the essential oils and absolutes that make up the aroma tones on our palette. Deep familiarity with them is the ground which can feed the roots of inspiration. We must not just get to know each but also the effects that they have on one another – some desirable, others not. We must know not just how each changes over time but how to influence these changes by judicious blending. It is all too easy to imagine one has taken the last step first and fall into the romantic identification with the ancient alchemists. Many mainstream perfumers have a reputation amongst their workmates for being a bit aloof and 'Prima Donna-ish' and the industry has by and large romanticised them. How to square this with certain celebrity fragrances would have Roudnitska turning in the grave. So what is it that we need and can it be taught or cultivated?

A good sense of smell is prerequisite but equally important is the ability to derive sensual pleasure from aromas. People who already have these capacities are the most likely to be attracted to perfumery. We need the ability to drop out of our conditioned layers of experience into our instinctual nature and have the naked immediacy of experiencing an odour on a non-verbal and non-judgemental level. This is using our nervous system to get an 'imprint' of each aroma. Language can then help us store this impression in our memory so that it is accessible. We should be able to go beyond like and dislike into naked experience. Meditation is, in my opinion, the best training to facilitate this dropping out of like and dislike into the naked immediacy of experience. In most people, smell becomes unconscious in early childhood because the majority of children are not encouraged to play using their noses. It is also no longer as important to us, as it was for our ancestors, in order to survive. To coax it back into consciousness a vocabulary is needed. Many people can smell very well but lack the descriptive ability, which is a combination of recognition and language. Imagine smell as a spectrum with an ultraviolet end, which is delicate, elusive, light, ethereal, diffusive and an infrared end which is heavy, earthy, and musky with every possible aroma in between. Language and guidance can help us to 'tune in' and differentiate more and more of this spectrum. I have been at tutored wine tastings where the tutor would say something like 'There is a delicate ginger biscuit quality' or something as specific. People mostly respond with 'Oh yes' i.e. they were able to detect it but unable to 'grasp it'. Very rarely is anybody unable to get it. With experience people learn to scan the entire range of the spectrum for themselves but each of us has 'blind spots' and we all have off days.

I think people who are exceptional cooks have only to become very familiar with the oils and understand a few principales in order to begin to blend. After that, the more experience the better. We must learn to play.

Creating a Fragrance

Any composition begins as a mental process so we start with conceptualising the nature of what it is we are trying to create. This might be following some parameters outlined by a client or it may originate entirely from within. Towards the end of the 19th Century the technique of making a fragrance according to the molecular weight of the constituents emerged. This method has since become standard and involves taking account of volatility when deciding upon the structure of a composition. In accordance with this method, each fragrance will comprise of top notes, middle notes and base notes. Over time, the most volatile (top notes) evaporate soonest and the least volatile (base notes) with much higher boiling points will stay on the skin for the greatest length of time. If a composition is overweight in top notes it will vanish very quickly and may be completely gone in a few minutes. If a composition is overweight in base notes it may last for days but will be difficult to detect. In a balanced composition the top notes, which provide the initial impression, should last for some minutes, the middle notes for at least a couple of hours and the base notes or dry away should be discernible for a few more hours or even longer. Most base notes act as fixatives by raising the boiling point of middle and top notes, making them last longer. The top and body notes bring some lift to the base notes. There have been several attempts to define precisely the proportions of each. We need to do this as a starting point, as it gives some measure but it will differ with fragrance type and desired effect. As a rule of thumb the base notes should comprise between 30% and 50% of the total blend. The remaining 70% to 50% can be divided up equally or slanted to favour lift (top notes) or intimacy (body notes).

I have my conceptual tool i.e. thinking about a fragrance in terms of *heart, nuance and intrigue*® very useful in this process. The heart is the body of the fragrance, its main theme. Nuance is provided by complimentary smell groups in order to make the heart more interesting and complex. Finally, intrigue is provided by unexpected, even dissonant notes, which invite curiosity by not being obvious. If you imagine the infrared/ultraviolet spectrum of top, middle and base as a vertical axis and if we combine the use of *heart, nuance and intrigue*® as a horizontal axis, we have a three dimensional model to aid conception.

A client presents us with a brief. They want a fragrance based on osmanthus which they love, having just smelled it. This is going to be the heart of their fragrance. Even if we are going to make a soliflor (single flower) fragrance we need more than just the single flower. By really 'listening' to the aroma of osmanthus we can get clues about what the nuance and intrigue might be. It is definitely floral – sweet, soft, warm, delicate, jasmine-like with hints of plum and dried fruit. You may also notice a similarity to mimosa in terms of a soft green back note and some slight waxy characteristics. We can enhance any of these characteristics by using other compatible oils, which have them in more prominence. Because of the inclusion of 'edible' notes and a light freshness in the floral quality, I am also inclined to think citrus. This would be discussed with the client during the consultation to try and define more and more precisely what it is about osmanthus that they love and other aromas they might want combined.

After some musing I may settle for something like the following as a starting point. ***Heart*** – osmanthus floral, ***Nuance*** – other florals, green notes, citrus, ***Intrigue*** – spices and herbs. At this point I may start making notes of what I intend to put into the composition. Experience tells me that so far there is not much evidence of base notes to act as fixatives to compound this; the client was not particularly keen on any of those heavier oils which would provide that function. The list I wrote looked like this:

Osmanthus
Mimosa
Jasmine
Rose Abs Maroc
Ylang Abs
Violet Leaf Abs.

This first group will provide the floral heart of the fragrance. Later, I will decide by a combination of experience and actual blending of the proportions. Small amounts of jasmine, rose and ylang always work well to give some substance but they must never be so much that they overwhelm the main effect which we are after – in this case osmanthus. Violet leaf absolute is included for the subtle greenness it brings and mimosa because it has a considerable overlap in odour profile with osmanthus. By including mimosa we are much more likely to get the feel of one harmonious floral scent. Never forget that you can always add more of something but it is impossible to take something out.

Lavender Abs
Coriander
Angelica
Clary Sage Abs
Thyme Abs
Lemon Myrtle

Lavender will marry the floral heart with the herbs as its odour profile naturally has both aspects. Coriander and angelica are included for effect and lift. Clary sage absolute will act as a fixative and with the thyme absolute add further depth, complexity and a hint of the Mediterranean sun. Lemon myrtle will marry the herbal notes with the citrus oils.

Litsea Cubeba
Grapefruit
Lime
Green Mandarin
Mint Abs.

Litsea cubeba has a distinctive lemony body, which is made more complex with grapefruit, green mandarin and a hint of lime before being freshened, lifted and greened by the mint abs. Experience tells me that the oils above are going to need fixing but I want to avoid heavy musky type fixatives as this will destroy the subtle delicacy of the osmanthus.

Benzoin
Tonka Bean
Labdanum
Frankincense
Vetivert Bourbon

There are many balsamic fixatives and these

can be very subtle and delicate so they do not interfere too much with the more ethereal aromas of the florals. On this occasion I have chosen benzoin, tonka bean abs and labdanum. Frankincense works not only as a superior fixative – it also helps to lighten the others in the blend. Vetivert Bourbon is included because it is a superior fixative with a distinctive green, earthy quality. Notice that we have green on each level – in the osmanthus, mimosa, violet leaf in the heart; in the herbs – angelica, thyme abs, clary sage abs; in the citrus – lime, green mandarin and, of course, mint abs. All this green is anchored by the green in the vetivert Bourbon. A good composition should be beautiful, seamless, complex, intriguing and work by fulfilling its function in terms of tenacity. It is all about proportion. After finalising the proportions of the above I decided to be bold and add some more intrigue and depth.

Tobacco Abs.
Vanilla Abs
Cocoa Abs.

The tobacco leaf abs brings some mysterious smoky notes and I decided to marry this into the balsamics by using the mother of all balsamics – vanilla abs and by way of a wild card, cocoa abs. A botanical musk fixative was also used at 5% of the scent content – not 5% of total volume. I am not going to disclose the exact proportions but will say there is more osmanthus in the blend than any other single ingredient. If osmanthus is the soloist then all the other oils in the orchestra support the soloist. It should not be a jam session amongst competing egomaniacal prima donnas.

Vanilla is a beautiful addition to many fragrances but caution is needed. It is one of a few absolutes that is not only very tenacious but its odour profile does not change much over time. In other words, it will easily dominate. This perfume is one of our house fragrances, which we call Kuan Yin to acknowledge the Chinese ancestry of osmanthus. Having named the perfume after Kuan Yin it then seemed appropriate to add some pink lotus absolute. Kuan Yin is a female manifestation of the compassion principle which appears in androgynous form in Tibet and India. In every Chinese Buddhist temple there is a shrine to Kuan Yin and it is usually adorned with pink lotus blooms.

The importance of precise record keeping cannot be overemphasised. It is an enormous aid to learning. There is absolutely no point in creating something amazing if we can't remember how we did it or repeat it. Using ratios is the most effective method as a unit of 1 can be one drop or one tonne. Assuming a simple floral blend that contains the following :-

Osmanthus	5
Mimosa	2
Jasmine	1
Rose Abs Maroc	1
Ylang Abs	0.5

Violet Leaf Abs.	0.3
Total	**9.8**

Blend using accurate measuring equipment – a 1ml pipette can measure down to 1/100 of 1ml. Make a small amount and only when you are happy with the blend add up the ratio parts as shown above. Now supposing you need to make 50 mls of the above blend. Subtract 8% (being the amount of water we are going to add later) from the desired quantity or take 92% of the desired amount. Either way we want 46mls. We divide 46 mls by 9.8 being the total of the ratios which gives us 4.69. Now simply multiply each of the ratio quantities by 4.69 and blend in the resulting quantities directly into a blending bottle. Add 4 mls (being 8%) of spring water. Please note that freshly blended fragrances take time to marry and mature. Using tinctures speeds this process up because each has already married with the alcohol base. Finished compositions should be left for at least a week at room temperature before chill filtering as described below.

After a week at room temperature, add a quarter teaspoon of fuller's earth and mix thoroughly and place the bottle upright in the fridge overnight. Chilling the blend in the fridge solidifies the wax content and the tiny particles of fuller's earth bind with smaller particles in the perfume and make them heavy enough to fall out of suspension.

The next day, without shaking, carefully pour the blend through a perfume grade filter. The sludge in the bottom, consisting of wax, fuller's earth and any stray plant material, can be poured out last into the funnel and left to drain slowly to avoid wastage. You will now have a crystal clear fragrance, which will not go cloudy again, even in a very cold bathroom. If you have used strong tinctures you will now have a concentrated fragrance, which you can dilute further using aged alcohol to get the desired strength.

SEVEN

Using Natural Raw Materials

Botanical raw materials in natural perfumery attempt to get as close as possible to the smell of the donor plant. Concretes, absolutes and essential oils are the three most common forms in which these smells are captured. Concretes are traditionally made when the heat from steam distillation would adversely affect the odour. The plant material is macerated in one of a number of volatile solvents, which causes the absolute and much of the wax (stearoptene) to dissolve. After filtration the solvent is removed by the application of gentle warmth. Having a very low boiling point, it evaporates easily leaving behind the concrete, which is a mixture of absolute and wax. To turn a concrete into an absolute, pure alcohol is used. As the absolute is completely soluble in alcohol and the wax only partially, it is easy to separate the two. Absolutes are the purest and most concentrated form of an essential oil. Both concretes and absolutes are closer to nature than an essential oil but can be much more difficult to work with. As well as all-important molecules of aroma, they can also contain very strong colours and can have very high wax contents. The natural colours form part of the charm and beauty of natural fragrances but the waxes make them difficult to handle. Many absolutes at room temperature are solid, making it impossible to use them or measure small quantities with any kind of precision. Benzoin resin in its natural state is like hard toffee, orris root concrete (also known as orris root butter) is solid like candle wax and many other concretes and absolutes resemble thick pastes.

To make them easy to work with, they can be made into mobile tinctures using alcohol. Like this, they can then be measured with ease down to one hundredth of 1 ml using a pipette. Fragrances are traditionally made in several strengths to reflect the function of each. Most quality perfumes have been launched as an extrait (please see table below) before coming onto the market in lesser concentrations at lower prices. The following table shows the approximate scent content of the different concentrations in alcohol and the name of each type.

Extrait	15% to 30% scent
Eau de parfum	8% to 15% scent
Eau de toilette	4 % to 8% scent
Eau de Cologne	3% to 5% scent
Eau fraiche	1% to 3 % scent

There are other advantages to using tinctures, apart from ease of measurability. The majority of tinctures improve with age and some benefit from very long term aging if protected from light and oxygen. As they mature, the smell of the alcohol becomes softer and softer and the tincture takes on more of the characteristics of the oil or absolute used in its manufacture. They magically seem to increase in strength. I recommend making up tinctures with essential oils as well as absolutes and concretes. If you are using delicate essential oils, like mandarin or bergamot, though they are easy-to-use because of their mobility, they are easily overpowered by the smell of fresh alcohol. However, if you make up tinctures and allow them to age a little, the desired effect in a blend can be achieved using smaller quantities than by adding them directly. Another advantage is that constituent parts of a composition marry more effectively and quickly using tinctures.

It is preferable to age alcohol before using it to make tinctures as this softens it, enabling it to marry more effectively with the most delicate of floral fragrances. To encourage the softening process it is usual to add in low dilution a blend of essential oils known for their fixation properties and other botanical extracts, making it gentler on the skin. The alcohol should be aged for at least three months before using it to make up tinctures. As an extrait is the strongest concentration of a fragrance, it makes good sense to make up and use tinctures of this strength.

I use extrait strength tinctures that are effectively single note fragrances containing 20% aromatic material in aged alcohol. It is a good idea to add some spring water to finished fragrances but the amount will vary with the composition. Water softens the alcohol and helps enhance the scent content so it is an important part of a finished fragrance. Alcohol and water will mix perfectly without going milky but once oil is introduced, a milky appearance will occur at certain concentrations. Remember that you can always add more water but you cannot take it out. As a rule of thumb it is safe to add 8% spring water to the final composition. If you want to add more than this 8% do so slowly, and in small increments, as the tipping point is arrived at suddenly. This is usually done before cold filtration as this will result in less wastage due to absorption by the filter paper. Once you have a finished fragrance it can be diluted further, in accordance with the table below, in order to arrive at the desired strength.

Eau de parfum 50% blended extraits and 50% aged alcohol and water.

Eau de toilette 40% blended extraits and 60 % aged alcohol and water.

Eau de Cologne 30% blended extraits and 70% aged alcohol and water.

Eau fraiche 20% blended extraits and 80% aged alcohol and water.

EIGHT

The A List

There are several ways of categorising natural aromatic raw materials and the success of each method is largely dependent on the intended final use. Categorising can be done by the part of the plant which renders the extract (wood, root, leaf, fruit etc), by key constituents (aldehyde, coumarin etc), by extraction method (steam, solvent, expression etc) or by smell category. As we are dealing with fragrance I have decided to use smell category. However, we do need some leeway as, for example, lavender could be categorised as floral or herby: burgeons de cassis could be fruity, animalistic (catty) or citrus and geranium could be floral, green or minty. Each scent is made up of layers and I have decided to classify by the main odour characteristic. Lavender absolute (middle note) I have categorised as floral, whereas lavender oil (top note) is herby. I hope pedants will forgive me for being somewhat subjective at times for the sake of neatness.

Citrus – *Crisp and Fresh*

Bergamot FCF

Production: Cold expression from peel of *Citrus Bergama.*
Origin: Sicily.
Use in Perfumery: extensively in classical eaux de colognes, chypre and fougère as a top note with fresh, sweet, rich, lemon, pepper, floral character which imparts lightness.
Safety: use only furanocoumarin free (FCF) as this constituent is phototoxic.
Comment: indispensable as a top note. The finest quality comes from Sicily.

Bitter Orange

Production: Cold expression from peel of *Citrus aurantium var amara.*
Origin: South America.
Use in Perfumery: Can be used in classical eaux de colognes, chypre and fougère compositions as a top note to impart a fresh, slightly bitter, orangey character with a pithy back note.
Safety: Do not exceed 1.4% of the pure oil in final blend or if using an extrait strength tincture at 20% dilution 7%.
Comment: More interesting and tenacious than sweet orange.

Grapefruit, Yellow

Production: Cold expression from peel of *Citrus paradisi.*
Origin: Israel, USA.
Use in Perfumery: Top note in citrus and cologne blends to impart fresh non-green sharpness, body and tenacity.
Safety: Do not exceed 4% in final blend.
Comment: Citrus oils are normally produced as a by-product of the juice industry. The trend in the market is to feed us more and more sugar so consumer preference is now for red grapefruit juice, consequently yellow grapefruits are becoming scarcer. The yellow oil costs more than the red for this reason alone. The nuketone content provides grapefruit with its 'bite' and even though this is a trace element the difference between 0.05% and 0.07% is fairly significant. The red grapefruit oil is much lower in nuketone than the yellow. I prefer the tang and 'bite' of the yellow to the fruitiness of the red, which can be invoked more economically by judicious blending of sweet orange, mandarin and lime.

Green Mandarin

Production: Cold expression from peel of unripe *Citrus reticulata.*
Origin: Sicily.
Use in Perfumery: As a light top note with fresh, sweet, green citrus character.
Safety: Normal usage.
Comment: Imparts interest to citrus blends and sharpness to floral blends. Mandarin is produced three times a year. The first time is when fruit naturally falls from the trees before it is ripe and is used to make the green mandarin. The fruit is later thinned by hand and these fruits go for yellow mandarin production and finally the ripe fruit is used to produce the red mandarin.

Lime Oil Distilled

Production: Steam distillation from the peel of *Citrus aurantifolia.*
Origin: Mexico.
Use in Perfumery: As a fresh, sweet, fruity, citrus lime top note in eaux de colognes.

Safety: This distilled oil is not phototoxic like the expressed variety.
Comment: Use with discretion, as it can easily overwhelm but used carefully it can provide a delicate lift to green florals.

Litsea Cubeba

Production: Steam distillation from ripe fruits of *Tetranthera polyantha.*
Origin: China, S.E. Asia.
Use in Perfumery: A sweet, fresh, lemony middle note with more intensity and tenacity than lemon. It smells more like lemon than lemon and adds body to citrus blends, though it can be somewhat coarse on its own.
Safety: Normal usage.
Comment: A good substitute for lemon, which has a tendency to oxidise and is phototoxic. The name cubeba comes from the shape of the fruits. It is known in China as may chang. See lemon myrtle.

Neroli Bigarade

Production: Steam distillation from blossoms of *Citrus aurantium var amara.*
Origin: Egypt.
Use in Perfumery: A light floral slightly bitter top note with herby green freshness, which leaves a trace of orange blossom in the dry out phase. Neroli softens citrus blends and imparts freshness and definition to florals. An important ingredient in classical eaux de colognes.
Safety: Normal usage
Comment: Invaluable versatile ingredient.

Petitgrain Oil Bigarade

Production: Steam distilled from the leaves and twigs of *Citrus aurantium var amara.*
Origin: Paraguay.
Use in Perfumery: Fresh orangey floral top note with bitter, herbal and a woody back note.
Safety: Normal usage.
Comment: Often used as a cheaper alternative to neroli but invaluable in its own right for the tenacity and body it brings to eaux de colognes and fougère blends.

Woody – *Soft yet Stable*

Cedarwood Atlas

Production: Steam distillation from woodchips of *Cedrus atlantica.*
Origin: Morocco.
Use in Perfumery: As for Virginian cedar but slightly heavier, with more body.
Safety: Normal usage.
Comment: A little more 'oily' than the Virginian. Both blend well with almost any other oil.

Cedarwood Virginian

Production: Steam distillation from woodchips of *Juniperus virginiana.*
Origin: USA.
Use in Perfumery: To impart a soft, woody top note with balsamic characteristics and a hint of earth to citrus, woody and floral blends. It can also act as a fixative.
Safety: Normal usage.
Comment: A number of cedar trees are used of the botanical species *Cedrus, Juniperus and Thuja.* Virginian or red cedar is the most widely used despite the fact that it is actually a juniper.

Cypress

Production: Steam distillation from leaves, twigs and woodchips of *Cupressus sempervirens.*
Origin: France.
Use in Perfumery: Light, woody top note with balsamic labdanum and smoky undertones.
Safety: Normal usage.
Comment: Versatile ingredient can help to fix citrus notes and balance light florals by adding some body.

Guaiacwood Oil

Production: Steam distillation from fine woodchips of *Bulnesia sarmienti.*
Origin: South America.
Use in Perfumery: Middle note, which is soft, sweet, balsamic and woody with a subtle rose- like character. Acts as an excellent fixative, especially for woody and floral type compositions. The cleanness of its aroma doesn't interfere with delicate florals.
Safety: Normal usage.
Comment: Also known as Champaca wood oil, Pao Santa, Palo balsamo and Paraguay Lignum. In its natural state Guaiacwood Oil is pale brown and has the consistency of a semi-solid paste.

Sandalwood Genuine

Production: Steam distillation from mature heartwood of *Santalum album.*
Origin: Mysore, New Caledonia.
Use in Perfumery: A soft, sweet, warm, woody balsamic and slightly fruity base note. Hugely versatile and without a doubt, by far the best wood oil available if you can get a reliable quality. One of a few outstanding fixatives and oils used for blending in many perfume types. Indispensible.
Safety: Normal usage.
Comment: Sandalwood oil improves with age in a tincture or in its natural state if properly stored by protecting from light, oxygen and extreme temperatures. It is well worth laying some down as prices can only keep rising. People are accustomed to paying high prices for absolutes but resist the price of genuine sandalwood. It priced itself out of commercial perfumery years ago but remains one of the most useful of all perfume materials. As such, I believe that it is worth every penny.

Balsamic – *Sweet and Warm*

Balsam of Peru

Production: Distilled from resinoid of *Myroxylon pereirae.*
Origin: South America.
Use in Perfumery: As a superior fixative in floral blends where it can impart an amber quality.
Safety: Do not exceed 2% of the pure oil in a blend.
Comment: Many balsams appear similar on first encounter and yet each is subtly different, as is the effect they can have in a blend. Only familiarity and experimentation will enable a perfumer to utilise their individual characteristics for fine-tuning of fragrances. The non-distilled oil is a sensitizer.

Balsam of Tolu

Production: Solvent extraction from resinoid of *Myroxylon toluifera.*
Origin: South America.
Use in Perfumery: Base note with rich, sweet, balsamic, floral quality with a hint of spice and fruit on a back note. Good fixative for heavier floral fragrances.
Safety: Normal usage.
Comment: Good choice for imparting warmth and body.

Benzoin Resin

Production: Solvent extraction from resinoid of *Styrax tokinensis.*
Origin: Thailand.
Use in Perfumery: Base note with sweet, balsamic, vanilla character which acts as a fixative. Especially good with light floral blends.
Safety: Normal usage.
Comment: Add in small increments as too much can overwhelm and obscure a blend's fragrance.

Frankincense

Production: Steam distillation from resinous tears of *Boswellia carterii.*
Origin: Arabian Peninsula.
Use in Perfumery: Fresh, resinous, balsamic, slightly green with a hint of lemon in the base note. A classy fixative and versatile blending ingredient.
Safety: Normal usage.
Comment: Highly valued in the ancient world. Frankincense tears were used as a currency and along with the spice and silk routes, there was also a frankincense route. Frankincense-derived wealth built Petra. This *Carteri* variety is vastly superior to the *Thurifera.* Not popular amongst lapsed Catholics, which can provoke insight into smell/learnt memory relationship.

Labdanum (Rock Rose, Cistus)

Production: Solvent extraction from resinous exudates of *Cistus ladaniferus.*

Origin: Mediterranean.

Use in Perfumery: A base note, which takes days to dry out. Sweet, rich, balsamic, amber character with warm, dry, woody back notes. Indispensable as a fixative.

Safety: Normal usage.

Comment: Herodotus (5th C BCE) observed Arabs combing the resin from the beards of their goats, which had grazed amongst labdanum bushes. It was also listed by him as one of the principal perfume ingredients brought from Arabia. Possibly the 'myrrh' referred to in the early chapters of the Bible. Often called amber by perfumers because it resembles ambergris and is used as the raw material for synthetic 'amber'. Listed as the main ingredient in 33% of modern quality fragrances, it blends well with almost anything. Essential component in chypre blends. If you pick only one balsamic fixative this has got to be it.

Myrrh

Production: Solvent extraction from oleo-gum-resin of *Commiphora molmol.*

Origin: Arabian Peninsula.

Use in Perfumery: Warm, spicy and at the limit of what could pass for balsamic. Good fixative for woody, chypre and oriental blends that imparts sweetness, depth and mystery.

Safety: Normal usage.

Comment: Goes well with opopanax, labdanum and tuberose.

Opopanax Resin

Production: Solvent extraction from oleo-gum-resin of *Commiphora erythroea.*

Origin: Arabian Peninsula.

Use in Perfumery: Fresh, warm, spicy, balsamic, resinous and slightly floral base note used a superior fixative in fine perfumery.

Safety: Normal usage.

Comment: A biblical balsam that goes well in oriental blends.

Tonka Bean Absolute

Production: Solvent extraction from dried beans of *Dipteryx odorata.*

Origin: South America.

Use in Perfumery: Rich, sweet and warm with hints of vanilla herbs and hay. Delicate and subtle quality fixative for fine fragrance use.

Safety: Normal usage.

Comment: Unlike most of the other balsamics this is very light in colour. The absolute is almost pure coumarin and was used as a source of coumarin until it could be synthesised more cheaply.

Vanilla Absolute

Production: Solvent extraction from crystals that form on cured beans of the orchid *Vanilla planifolia.*

Origin: Madagascar.
Use in Perfumery: Base note with sweet, rich, warm, vanilla character which blends beautifully with heavier floral and oriental compositions.
Safety: Normal usage.
Comment: It is one of a small number of fixatives that holds its odour profile on a smelling strip over many days. Associated by many people with synthetic vanillin and bubble gum notes that we're told 'celebritneys' smell of. The real thing is rich, warm, deep, mysterious, heady and incredibly sexy. It dances all night with jasmine, patchouli, frankincense and sandalwood. Greening vanilla with violet leaf and warming with celery or caraway seed makes it sophisticated and intimate.

Floral – *Delicate or Intense but Always Beautiful*

Boronia Absolute

Production: Solvent extraction from fresh flower spikes of *Boronia megastigma.*
Origin: Tasmania/Australia.
Use in Perfumery: Its top note is fresh but the body is extraordinarily warm and rich in violet, lily, freesia notes against a beautifully soft green back note.
Safety: Normal usage.
Comment: The concrete was exhibited at the British Empire Exhibition of 1924 yet has remained obscure until recently. It has been used as a flavour in confectionery. It has become extremely rare as a result of gaining iconic status amongst natural perfumers. Due to the scarcity of supply it is unfortunately reserved for our house perfumes and personal fragrance service.

Geranium Bourbon

Production: Steam distillation from leaves and branches of *Pelargonium graveolens.*
Origin: Réunion, formerly known as Bourbon.
Use in Perfumery: A fresh, rosy middle note with a slightly green, minty quality. Very useful for bolstering rose, if not allowed to dominate. It can also be used to freshen up and bring depth to other floral notes.
Safety: Normal usage.
Comment: Bourbon is indisputably the premium quality geranium oil.

Genet Absolute (Spanish Broom)

Production: Solvent extraction from very fresh flowers of *Spartium junceum.*
Origin: France.
Use in Perfumery: Sweet, fresh, delicate floral

with hints of hay. Excellent for softening intense floral blends and warming citrus.
Safety: Normal usage.
Comment: Grown in southern France and Spain since the 16th C as a perfume ingredient. The flowers are similar in appearance to those of the sweet pea to which it is related. The Plantagenets named themselves after this plant (*Planta genet*).

Immortelle Absolute

Production: Solvent extraction from fresh petals or concrete of *Helichrysum angustifolium.*
Origin: France.
Use in Perfumery: Floral, sweet and woody, with hints of herb, honey and hay. Base note blender in floral compositions. Lovely in masculine type chypre, amber or fougère fragrances.
Safety. Normal usage.
Comment: Deserves to be much better known.

Jasmine Absolute – the King of flowers

Production: Solvent extraction from concrete of *Jasminum officinalis.*
Origin: Egypt.
Use in Perfumery: Traditionally used in the finest compositions with rose and neroli to provide a classical floral heart. Will enhance almost any feminine blend and in lower doses almost any masculine fragrance. Quite intense, heady, floral character with fruity, green back notes. Its long dry out period helps the persistence of other floral scents in a blend.
Safety: Normal usage.
Comment: Indispensable oil for the natural perfumer. Like vanilla, synthetically 'enhanced' jasmines are so prolific that many people don't like it until they come across the real thing, which has a depth and complexity that when used in the right proportions is magical. Remains inimitable.

Jasmine Sambac Absolute

Production: Solvent extraction from concrete of *Jasminum sambac.*
Origin: India, China.
Use in Perfumery: Sweet, fresh, light, white floral and lily-like with a delicate, ethereal, soft, green backnote. Like its cousin above a versatile, classy, floral middle note. Also known as Arabian or sometimes Tuscan jasmine. The English name is derived from the Arabic zanbaq and has a long history of fragrance use in India where the plant is known as chameli and the oil as motia.
Safety: Normal usage.
Comment: I have been offered the absolute many times in India but never encountered one that justified the asking price (it is usually more expensive than *J.officinalis* or *J.grandiflorum*). However , one of my Chinese suppliers sent me

a sample that had the tingle factor. It reminded me of the smell inside a quality florist's shop. The top note has an elusive floral character partly reminiscent of bunches of freesias or lilies. It is too fresh to be heady, courtesy of the angelic, green back note. I sent a sample to a colleague from a French fragrance company. When I asked him for his opinion he said,'I want to lick it.'

Lavender Absolute

Production: Solvent extraction from flower heads of *Lavendula angustafolia.*
Origin: France.
Use in Perfumery: As a fresh, floral middle note in almost any blend. Its ability to marry floral, herbal and woody notes in a blend is incomparable. Fresh, floral lavender with backnotes of herb, wood and hay.
Safety: Normal usage.
Comment: The absolute is much more floral, deep and complex than the oil. Over familiarity and its popularity should not prevent its use; truly versatile, dark blue.

Linden Blossom Absolute

Production: Solvent extraction from dried flowers of *Tilea europea.*
Origin: France.
Use in Perfumery: Light, warm, citrus and floral with hints of beeswax and honey. Works well to impart green notes to floral blends and adds subtlety and warmth to citrus and chypre fragrances.
Safety: Normal usage.
Comment: Essential part of floral/citrus palette along with neroli.

Mimosa Absolute

Production: Solvent extraction from fresh flowers of *Acacia dealbata.*
Origin: France.
Use in Perfumery: Soft, sweet, floral and waxy top note with a hint of balsam and a light green back note. Excellent for lifting and as a marrying agent in many fragrance categories. Good for blends that require a delicate or subtle floral quality.
Safety: Normal usage.
Comment: Grown up floral – Floris *non polyana.*

Orange Flower Absolute

Production: Solvent extraction from fresh blossom of *Citrus aurantium var amara.*
Origin: Tunisia.
Use in Perfumery: As a fresh middle note providing a fragrant bouquet in many types of composition. Flexible enough to use in delicate and light floral blends or to add a rich, intense, heavy, green, orange blossom scent.
Safety: Normal usage.

Comment: Extremely versatile and a candidate to prove the 'less is more rule'. Blends beautifully with neroli and lavender absolute but brings out nuances in almost any other floral.

Orris Root Concrete

Production: Steam distilled from dried rhizomes of *Iris pallida* with a yield of 1-2 parts per 1000, effectively an essential oil, but solid at room temperature.
Origin: Italy.
Use in Perfumery: Another highly important perfume material. A top note reminiscent of violets but so delicate with warm, fruity, tenacious undertones. The real magic is the effect it has on other oils in a composition. It is an excellent fixative and has the power to amplify other notes in a fragrance.
Safety: Normal usage.
Comment: Orris root concrete – this is the premium orris product, also known as butter/ beurre due to its appearance. The plant is named after the Goddess of the rainbow and has been esteemed for centuries. The best is produced from three-year old dried rhizomes of *Iris pallida.* Quality and therefore price is determined by the irone content. This butter has an irone content of 16% and is the best quality that money can buy.

Osmanthus Absolute (Kwei Hwa, Mo Hsi)

Production: Solvent extraction from fresh flowers of *Osmanthus fragrans.*
Origin: France.
Use in Perfumery: Sweet, soft, warm, delicate, jasmine-like floral, with hints of plum and dried fruit. Another grown up floral, which adds interest and sophistication to fragrances. Blends well with mimosa and violet leaf.
Safety: Normal usage.
Comment: Flowers of an evergreen tree native to China and Japan. It surprises. Part of the beauty of blending naturals is the effect that oils have on each other. Experience means fewer surprises but nature usually has the last word. Recently, when working on a perfume, osmanthus produced completely unbidden delicate notes of peach blossom. Beautiful.

Pink Lotus Absolute

Production: Solvent extraction from fresh blooms of Nelumbo *nucifera.*
Origin: India.
Use in Perfumery: In floral compositions to impart fresh, floral, warm, rich and slightly heady notes. Blends well with quality green notes to produce exotic yet understated character.
Safety: Normal usage.
Comment: Chosen from several kinds of lotus.

We found that the pink lotus was the most consistent quality and had the most unique fragrance.

Rose Absolute Maroc (Rose de Mai)

Production: Solvent extraction from fresh petals of *Rosa centifolia.*
Origin: Morocco.
Use in Perfumery: As for rose otto, it can form the backbone of a blend or transform a lack lustre composition. It brings warmth, delicacy, smoothness, harmony and beauty. Again it will blend with almost anything.
Safety: Normal usage.
Comment: Wax Lyrical.

Rose Otto – The Queen of Flowers

Production: Distillation from fresh petals of *Rosa damascena.*
Origin: Bulgaria.
Use in Perfumery: Only limited by cost as it is so versatile that it can be used in almost any type of fragrance to impart rich, rosy, floral notes. A middle note of great tenacity, making it effective in small doses – a great harmoniser.
Safety: Normal usage.
Comment: Perfumers are divided on preference for Turkish or Bulgarian otto. Originally, the rose of Damascus was introduced to Bulgaria by a visiting Turkish merchant. Bulgaria is now the largest producer followed by Turkey. Cultivation and husbandry is labour intensive, which combined with extremely low yields and the fact that more than one distillation is needed accounts for the cost. Rose is unquestionably the single most important oil in perfumery.

Tuberose Absolute

Production: Solvent extraction from concrete of *Polyanthes tuberosa.*
Origin: France.
Use in Perfumery: Mainly used in sweet, heavier floral and oriental compositions. Small doses enhance light florals with body. Sweet, heavy, floral and balsamic, with slightly green, honey back note. Has been described as a 'well stocked garden at eventide.'
Safety: Normal usage.
Comment: Known as mistress of the night in India and Malaysia as the growing blooms get more intense after nightfall. The cut flowers are extracted by enfleurage because they continue to produce essential oil for 48 hours after being picked. Native to either Indonesia or Mexico and Central America. Highly valued by the Aztecs.

White Champac Absolute

Production: Solvent extraction from fresh flowers of *Michelia champaca.*

Origin: India.
Use in Perfumery: To impart powerful sweet, heady, velvety, floral character with hints of lily, hay and orange blossom. Versatile enough to produce delicate, soft, floral character or something approaching jasmine-like intensity.
Safety: Normal usage.
Comment: On special occasions in India and Thailand flowers are sometimes picked in the morning and woven into the hair in order to scent it. The flowers carry on producing oil for some hours after they have been picked. During the day they gradually open, but being indolic, seduction happens at night when they release their soft magic, which hangs invisible in the air. The genuine absolute is scarce.

Ylang Absolute

Production: Solvent extraction from freshly picked flowers of *Cananga odorata*.
Origin: Madagascar.
Use in Perfumery: To provide lift and as a harmoniser in heavy type floral blends. Tropical, floral quality with hints of fruit, medicine and spice with a slightly balsamic dry out. The absolute is softer than the oil and acts as a middle note.
Safety: Normal usage.
Comment: Extremely useful, especially in oriental compositions. Enhances most floral blends in small doses by bringing lightness. The cheap ylang oils are used as a flavour in fruity chewing gum and highly synthetic versions are responsible for the bubble gum note in modern mass produced perfumes. As Rumi says, without gold there could be no false coin. Another absolute, which can be used well below the level of conscious detection yet which still imparts valuable body, some lift and a harmonising effect.

Herbaceous – *Earth, Sun and Sea*

Clary Sage Absolute

Production: Solvent extraction from fresh *Salvia sclarea*.
Origin: France.
Use in Perfumery: Used as a fixative and also for its appealing sweet, light, herby, woody, amber warmth. The absolute is much warmer than the oil. Classically included in chypre, fougère, oriental and herbal compositions for its distinctive notes. Can be used in small doses in almost every type of blend.
Safety: Normal usage.
Comment: Extracted sclareol is used as a natural fixative.

Coriander

Production: Steam distillation from dried seeds of *Coriandrum sativum.*

Origin: France.
Use in Perfumery: A fresh top note useful with heavy florals and oriental type blends. Quite intense with notes of fresh, peppery, spicy, woody, floral with a green herb character. Brings freshness and intrigue.
Safety: Normal usage.
Comment: Use in moderation. Like many of the spices they bring their best when below the threshold of conscious detection.

Laurel Leaf Absolute

Production: solvent extraction from crushed leaves of *Laurus nobilis.*
Origin: Italy.
Use in Perfumery: More interesting than the oil. Fresh, warm, green, slightly basil-like with hints of spice. Imparts quality herbal notes, without the camphor usually found in the oil. Blends beautifully with citrus, spice and wood.
Safety: Normal usage.
Comment: Use of laurel leaf oil is voluntarily restricted by some fragrance houses. The absolute is preferable.

High Altitude Lavender oil

Production: Steam distillation from fresh high altitude *Lavendula angustafolia.*
Origin: France.
Use in Perfumery: Truly versatile top note. Good quality lavender should have real body with sweet, fresh, light, fruity top notes giving way to a strong, herbal, lavender, floral, woody body. Use for marrying wood and herb with floral notes.
Safety: Normal usage.
Comment: Carefully chosen from top high altitude qualities. Oil produced from high grown plants has a higher ester content (typically 10% more) than oil made from its siblings grown nearer sea level. The esters are responsible for the floral character in the oil making high altitude lavender the natural choice for perfume use.

Lemon Myrtle

Production: Steam distillation from partly dried *Myrtus citriadora.*
Origin: Spain.
Use in Perfumery: Another warm Mediterranean herbal, woody oil with strong lemon character. Adds freshness to top notes and character to citrus blends. Try with thyme absolute in colognes.
Safety: Normal usage.
Comment: Lemon oil has the tendency to oxidise quite quickly so use this instead. Also see *litsea cubeba*.

Roman Chamomile Absolute

Production: Solvent extraction from florets of *Anthemis nobilis.*
Origin: France.

Use in Perfumery: This sweet, warm, fruity, herbal absolute is also very versatile. An excellent marrying agent, but also produces warmth to woody accords and lift to florals.
Safety: Normal usage.
Comment: Similar odour profile to quality oil but more warmth and depth.

Thyme Absolute

Production: Solvent extraction from partly dried *Thymus vulgaris.*
Origin: France.
Use in Perfumery: The oil is used in small doses to impart fresh, woody, herby top notes but the absolute brings Mediterranean sunshine and body – a warm, herbal, woody breeze with hints of spice and tobacco in the dry out.
Safety: Normal usage.
Comment: If you are new to herbal absolutes and you wish to try one, choose this. Very versatile. Goes well with woody, citrus and floral blends.

Spicy – *Unexpected, Edgy, Intriguing*

Black Pepper

Production: Steam distillation from unripe berries of *Piper nigrum.*
Origin: India.
Use in Perfumery: Top note. Used for its warm, dry, spicy, woody note that produces special effects.
Safety: Normal usage.
Comment: Another one to go easy with.

Caraway Seed

Production: Steam distillation from seeds of *Carum carvi.*
Origin: France.
Use in Perfumery: Same umbellifers family as celery seed and has similar uses. However, caraway is much warmer and spicy; it blends beautifully with jasmine and in oriental type blends.
Safety: Normal usage.
Comment: An oil well worth getting to know.

Carrot Seed

Production: Steam distillations from dried seeds of *Daucus carota.*
Origin: France.
Use in Perfumery: In traces for its sweet, fresh, woody, earthy top note and to bring lift to the green classics, Oriental and floral compositions.
Safety: Normal usage.
Comment: Like the other seed oils they have an'outdoorsy'quality and are useful in daytime blends.

Celery Seed

Production: Steam distillation from crushed seeds of *Apium graveolens.*
Origin: France.
Use in Perfumery: A useful base note, which brings warmth to heavy florals. The oil is spicy, warm and rich with a long dry out showing little change. Very tenacious.
Safety: Normal usage.
Comment: Less is more especially when used with the lighter florals. Can also add intrigue to the balsams.

Cinnamon Leaf

Production: Steam distillation from leaves of *Cinnamomum zeylanicum.*
Origin: Sri Lanka.
Use in Perfumery: In minute doses for its sweet, warm, spicy, fruit character. Used particularly in floral and oriental blends.
Safety: Do not exceed 0.5% in a composition. Avoid using cinnamon bark oil.
Comment: Avoid the oil from the bark. This is very useful if you take it easy. A tad too much and you're into the pot pourri zone. If you like pot-pourri type fragrances you are reading the wrong book.

Clove Bud

Production: Distillation from sun dried unopened flower buds of *Eugenia caryophyllata.*
Origin: Zanzibar.
Use in Perfumery: In very small doses to impart warmth and richness to almost any blend. Fresh, fruity, sweet, rich, spicy, woody with balsamic undertone. Often used in floral compositions.
Safety: Normal usage.
Comment: The genuine bud oil is the only one to use in perfumery. It has a smooth richness and warmth completely lacking in the cheaper stem and leaf oils. The higher cost is not just a question of yield. The flower buds are removed from the stem by hand, which is very labour intensive. Eugenol, a key constituent, is also found in carnation absolute which makes clove bud oil a natural choice to use in many floral blends.

Fenugreek

Production: Steam distillation from seeds of *Trigonella foenum-graecum.*
Origin: France.
Use in Perfumery: Intrigue, intrigue and intrigue. Initial impression is overwhelmingly of curry, but stay with it and a warm walnut like odour appears which adds a rich tone to most blends if not overdone. Used by the early Arabs in their perfumes.
Safety: Normal usage.
Comment: Try blending a minute quantity with your favourite floral or wood. *Foenum-graecum* means 'Greek hay', so called because fenugreek seeds were used by the ancient Greeks to scent inferior hay.

Nutmeg

Production: Steam distillation from the seeds of *Myristica fragrans.*
Origin: Indonesia.
Use in Perfumery: To add warmth and intrigue. Extensively used especially in men's fragrances and in smaller amount in many other blends. The oil has a fresh, light, warm, sweet and woody odour with spicy undertones.
Safety: Do not exceed 0.5% of the pure oil in a composition.
Comment: Like many of the spices, they bring their best when below the threshold of conscious detection.

Agrestic – *Down on the Farm*

Beeswax Absolute

Production: Solvent extraction from honeycombed wax propolis of *Apis mellifera L*
Origin: Italy.
Use in Perfumery: Rich, warm, honeyed with soft green back notes of hay.
Safety: Normal usage but don't forget your pipe when raiding the hive.
Comment: Highly underrated fixative which is as versatile as guaiacwood.

Galbanum Resinoid

Production: Natural resin exuded by *Ferula galbaniflua.*
Origin: Iran.
Use in Perfumery: The resinoid is a base note, which is used as a fixative in any composition with green notes. It can also be used to freshen up the base notes in heavy oriental type compositions. Green, sharp, spicy, balsamic notes mask a slightly floral, earthy agrestic body.
Safety: Normal usage.
Comment: A giant fennel whose resin is used as a medicine in Iran. The resinoid has traditionally been blended with opopanax in old Arabian perfumery.

Galbanum Oil

Production: Steam distillation from the resinoid of *Ferula galbaniflua.*
Origin: Turkey.
Use in Perfumery: Spicy, green and leaf like top note, used in small doses to contribute its character to the green classics. It can also be used to bring intrigue to other oils with natural greenness like violet leaf and geranium.
Safety: Normal usage.
Comment: Not so interesting on its own, but none the less very much a part of the green palette because of the effect it has on other oils.

Hay Absolute

Production: Solvent extraction from dried *Hierochloe alpina.*
Origin: Italy.
Use in Perfumery: Very seldom used in mainstream perfumery because synthetic coumarin, which has a hay-like odour, is much cheaper. This absolute is warm, sweet, rich, green and yes, hay-like. It can lighten intense florals, warm citrus and introduce green notes to almost any blend.
Safety: Normal usage.
Comment: Perhaps a contender for a happy smell. We have yet come across anyone who suffers from hay fever being adversely affected by the absolute.

Tobacco Leaf Absolute

Production: Solvent extraction from semi-dried *Nicotianum tabacum.*
Origin: France.
Use in Perfumery: Rich, warm, amber with greenish hue and also deep, dark and mysterious. The synthetic versions used in mainstream perfumery cannot get anywhere near this depth. Lovely with citrus, especially lime and linden blossom. Imparts warmth and depth to florals.
Safety: Normal usage.
Comment: This and oakmoss are contenders for the most butch oils.

Vetivert Bourbon

Production: Steam distillation from roots of *Vetivera zizanoides.*
Origin: Réunion formerly known as Bourbon.
Use in Perfumery: Invaluable as a fixative. It has a sweet, earthy, woody, green character that remains the same over many days on a strip. Its woody note is inimitable in the green classics, woody, oriental and floral blends.
Safety: Normal usage.
Comment: The Bourbon is the premium quality, being much smoother and deeper than more common grade vetivert from Java.

Green – *Very Leafy*

Violet Leaf Absolute

Production: Solvent extraction from concrete of *Viola odorata.*
Origin: France.
Use in Perfumery: Traditionally in the green classics but its green, woody, floral, earthy character can be used in small doses to impart body and intrigue to all the quality florals. A middle note that certainly knows how to bring ylang absolute down to earth. Compliments osmanthus and mimosa beautifully.
Safety: Normal usage.
Comment: Very dark green in colour. The obvious combination is with orris concrete, but try it with lavender absolute, too.

Mossy – *If You Go Down To The Woods*

Oakmoss Absolute

Production: Solvent extraction from dried lichen *Evernia prunastri* collected from the bark of oak trees.
Origin: France.
Use in Perfumery: For richness, complexity, fixation and its earthy, woody scent with hints of musk and smoked amber. Hugely important, due to its unique odour profile and especially used for chypre and fougère compositions but it blends beautifully with most oils.
Safety: Do not exceed 0.1% of the pure oil in final blend.
Comment: Imported by the ancient Egyptians from the Greeks and used to leaven and flavour bread. A victim of modern sensibility and Euro legislation, despite the centuries of use as a highly valued perfume ingredient. If you are a chypre fan you can bolster a low dose of oak moss absolute with tobacco leaf absolute and any or all of the following:- labdanum, clary sage absolute, thyme absolute, blackcurrant bud absolute, violet leaf absolute, seaweed absolute, linden blossom absolute and mint absolute. Dead butch.

Minty – *Fresh Green, Spring Breeze*

Mint Absolute

Production: Solvent extraction from leaves and stem of *Mentha piperita.*
Origin: France.
Use in Perfumery: To impart fresh cool green notes or in small doses to lift heavier blends, especially florals and the green classics.
Safety: Normal usage.
Comment: Delighted to have found a source for this. It completely lacks the sharp harsh notes of even the best peppermint or spearmint. This is soft and round; it has much more the quality of garden mint – the same kind of minty note found in good geranium.

Marine – *Lets Go Surfing Now*

Seaweed Absolute

Production: Solvent extraction from dried *Fucus vesiculosus.*
Origin: French concrete processed to an absolute in Italy.
Use in Perfumery: For green, salty, evocative oceanic effect in all the green classics and for adding intrigue to many other types of blend.

Safety: Normal usage.
Comment: There are so many kinds of seaweed and not many are suitable for fragrance use. This one took some finding and it really has the sea in it. Not many marine notes available to the natural perfumer but the 'outdoorsy' mainstream fragrance market is popular with aspiring 'ruffty tuffties'.

Mavericks – *Oddballs That Can Make The Party*

Blackcurrant Bud Absolute

Production: Solvent extraction from flower buds of *Ribes nigrum.*
Origin: France.
Use in Perfumery: Is it citrus? Is it fruity? Is it minty? Is it catty? Is it green? Well yes, we think so. Imparts very interesting fruity character to wide range of blends.
Safety: Normal usage.
Comment: Versatile as it is elusive.

Cocoa Absolute

Production: Solvent extracted from the fruit and seeds of *Theobroma cacao.*
Origin: Venezuela.
Use in Perfumery: One of the so-called edibles. The absolute is rich, warm, sweet, balsamic and chocolate like, with fixative properties. Can be used to impart exotic effects.
Safety: Normal usage.
Comment: A common reaction to this is, 'like the smell, but not sure if I want to smell of it'. If it is blended properly you won't. Very dark brown.

Coffee Absolute

Production: Solvent extraction from roasted berries of *Coffea arabica.*
Origin: South America.
Use in Perfumery: Intrigue with deep, rich, roasted, exotic, warm, earthy quality.
Safety: Normal usage.
Comment: Extremely low yielding, which accounts for its high price.

Green Cognac Absolute

Production: Distilled from the lees of wine (fermented juice of *Vitus vinifera)* used for cognac production.
Origin: France.
Use in Perfumery: For special effects – an ethereal, warm, spicy nuance. Small doses produce a fruity grape aroma. I prefer the green to the white as it has more interest in its aroma.

Safety: Normal usage.
Comment: Tobacco, cognac, leather and coffee – it has been tried.

Patchouli

Production: Steam distillation from dried leaves of *Pogostemom patchouli.*
Origin: Indonesia.
Use in Perfumery: Inimitable. Used so extensively, according to one perfumer, that it is impossible to specify its field of application. Sweet, extremely rich, spicy, woody, balsamic, slightly floral and extremely tenacious. A great fixative used in small doses in any blend or as a fundamental note in orientals and heavy florals.
Safety: Normal usage.
Comment: The best patchouli should have an ethereal-floral character to its top note that is almost wine-like. One of several oils that improves with age, becoming more fruity, rounded and elusive. It will keep for decades if stored properly. People who dislike patchouli usually have associations with it that puts them off. Reluctant to shake off its hippie, don't wash or 'me smell of dope?' image. Absolutely one of the most useful of all essential oils in perfumery. Goes with everything, including people who don't like it.

Appendix

Explanation of Trace, Report and Certificate

Rose Maroc Gas Liquid Chromatography (GLC) Trace.

Gas chromatography is used to analyse volatile compounds. In order to understand how it works imagine a long, small diameter tube. A minute sample of the oil to be analysed is introduced to one end of the tube and is shunted along the tube by gas under pressure. The application of heat encourages the oil's tendency to vaporise. Natural aromatic oils are complex mixtures of molecules and some constituents in the oil are more volatile than others. The temperature is gradually increased to encourage the less volatile molecules to vaporise. The most volatile constituent will vaporise first, followed by the second and so on until the very last one goes puff. If the tube, which is called the column, is very long (30 metres) and the temperature inside is constant throughout the length then the first constituent to vaporise will be the first constituent to emerge from the other end. The longer the tube, the greater the time difference between the vaporising of a particular constituent and its emergence from the other end of the column. Constituents of the same kind emerge in a group and each group of molecules is measured by computer. The result is presented in the form of a trace on a graph which gives a visual odour profile.

The vertical axis shows retention time, which begins when the oil is introduced to the column. Each group of vaporised molecules is represented by a 'peak' and the bigger the peak the more molecules of that constituent are present. The horizontal axis shows the quantity. The time lag between one constituent vaporising and the next is shown by a flat line i.e. nothing is vaporising. The trace needs interpreting by a specialist and you can see that the name of the corresponding constituent has been written on the major peaks (page 88). The trace is usually presented in the form of a table showing the percentage of major constituents. Eucalyptus oil is simple and can be over 90% one constituent; for tea tree oil two key constituents are used as indicators of quality. It is not just the percentage but their relationship is important, too. In tea tree, for example,, one of the major constituents is inversely proportional to another. In complex oils like rose which has over 400 constituents, only a small number are used for quality assessment.

The certificate of analysis from Bulgaria shows the 'Tupical' percentage content of major constituents. All of those constituents are available in synthesised form and if you blended synthetic counterparts in the same proportion, you would naturally assume that the odour profile would be similar to that of natural rose. You would be very wrong indeed because naturals have a complexity that in many cases defy imitation due to the many trace elements. It is possible, however, to imitate synthetics using synthetics and this is how copycat fragrances are made. Notice that phenyl ethyl alcohol is present at 62.44%. Synthetic phenyl ethyl alcohol in bulk costs a few pounds a kilo and is used as a blender and extender to produce cheap rose smells. The better qualities of rose fragrances will have an increasing amount of natural rose blended with the aroma chemicals.

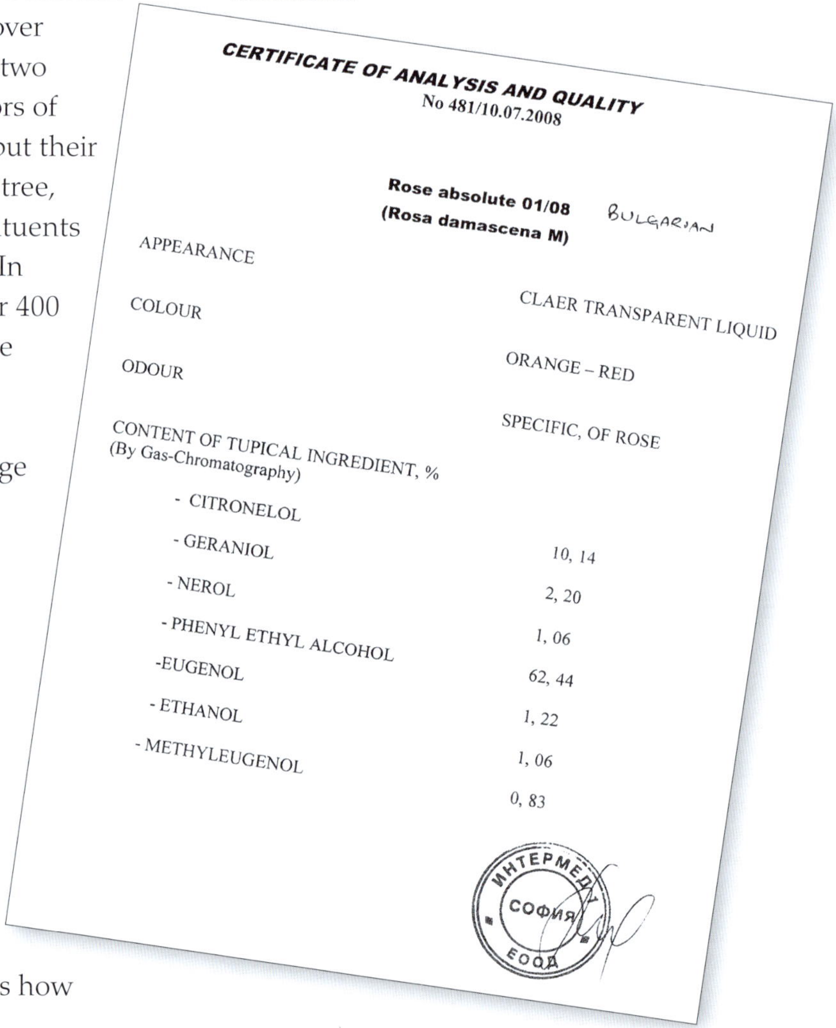

CERTIFICATE OF ANALYSIS AND QUALITY
No 481/10.07.2008

Rose absolute 01/08
(Rosa damascena M) BULGARIAN

APPEARANCE	CLAER TRANSPARENT LIQUID
COLOUR	ORANGE – RED
ODOUR	SPECIFIC, OF ROSE
CONTENT OF TUPICAL INGREDIENT, % (By Gas-Chromatography)	
- CITRONELOL	10, 14
- GERANIOL	2, 20
- NEROL	1, 06
- PHENYL ETHYL ALCOHOL	62, 44
-EUGENOL	1, 22
- ETHANOL	1, 06
- METHYLEUGENOL	0, 83

ИНТЕРМЕД 1 СОФИЯ ЕООД

ROSE MOROCCO ABSOLUTE AT 158

AROUK 303

Batch n° : SDHE/06/41/0062

Software Version	: 6.2.1.0 104:0104	Date	: 10/12/2006 1:02:38 PM
Operator	: pc9	Sample Name	: ABS ROSE MAROC
Sample Number	: 157	Study	:
AutoSampler	: BUILT-IN	Rack/Vial	:
Instrument Name	: AUTOSYSTEM XL	Channel	: A
Instrument Serial #	: 610N7102801	A/D mV Range	: 1000
Delay Time	: 0.00 min	End Time	: 122.51 min
Sampling Rate	: 1.5625 pts/s		
Sample Volume	: 1.000000 ul	Area Reject	: 0.000000
Sample Amount	: 1.0000	Dilution Factor	: 1.00
Data Acquisition Time	: 10/12/2006 7:12:34 AM	Cycle	: 9

Raw Data File : E:\TCWS\autoxl\data\ABSROSEMAROCA80.raw
Result File : E:\TCWS\autoxl\data\ABSROSEMAROCA80-20061012-130235.rst
Inst Method : e:\tcws\autoxl\methodes\lavlong from E:\TCWS\autoxl\data\ABSROSEMAROCA80.raw
Proc Method : e:\tcws\autoxl\methodes\lavlong.mth from E:\TCWS\autoxl\data\ABSROSEMAROCA80-20061012-130235.rst
Calib Method : e:\tcws\autoxl\methodes\lavlong.mth from E:\TCWS\autoxl\data\ABSROSEMAROCA80-20061012-130235.rst
Report Format File: e:\tcws\autoxl\methodes\lavpurm.rpt
Sequence File : E:\TCWS\autoxl\sequences\LAVPURM.seq

DEFAULT REPORT

Peak #	Time [min]	Area [µV·s]	Height [µV]	Area [%]	Norm. Area [%]	BL	Area/Height [s]
1	8.561	2865.20	536.80	0.02	0.02	BB	5.3376
2	8.921	7286.29	1104.95	0.06	0.06	BB	6.5943
3	11.972	11925.26	1735.05	0.09	0.09	BB	6.8732
4	13.849	5874.76	1283.11	0.05	0.05	BB	4.5785
5	14.323	6243.86	1182.19	0.05	0.05	BB	5.2816
6	15.139	3938.19	814.09	0.03	0.03	BB	4.8375
7	15.654	139099.92	17237.14	1.09	1.09	BV	8.0698
8	16.469	42017.59	7544.62	0.33	0.33	VB	5.5692
9	18.081	1751.09	309.69	0.01	0.01	BB	5.6544
10	18.368	3158.78	463.70	0.02	0.02	BB	6.8121
11	20.783	8942872.05	421899.92	70.04	70.04	BE	21.1967
12	21.139	57771.74	2116.05	0.45	0.45	EB	27.3017
13	22.159	1776.93	353.60	0.01	0.01	BB	5.0253
14	22.604	3753.00	687.09	0.03	0.03	BB	5.4621
15	24.155	13724.04	2424.15	0.11	0.11	BB	5.6614
16	25.246	4572.32	764.73	0.04	0.04	BB	5.9790
17	25.960	6707.99	1043.74	0.05	0.05	BV	6.4269
18	26.152	8148.86	1425.43	0.06	0.06	VV	5.7168
19	26.413	2607.47	395.21	0.02	0.02	VB	6.5976
20	28.558	894452.33	126615.63	7.01	7.01	BB	7.0643
21	29.550	34254.47	5955.67	0.27	0.27	BB	5.7516
22	30.194	421395.73	66905.14	3.30	3.30	BV	6.2984
23	30.483	35934.96	5922.33	0.28	0.28	VV	6.0677
24	30.692	15956.88	2461.26	0.12	0.12	VB	6.4832
25	31.643	3220.52	521.57	0.03	0.03	BB	6.1747
26	32.585	6262.01	827.71	0.05	0.05	BB	7.5655
27	33.149	1560.85	261.95	0.01	0.01	BB	5.9586
28	35.059	1490.74	254.59	0.01	0.01	BB	5.8555
29	36.493	114526.81	18902.97	0.90	0.90	BV	6.0587
30	36.841	18296.28	2443.08	0.14	0.14	VB	7.4890
31	37.417	3149.64	461.09	0.02	0.02	BB	6.8308
32	38.612	19935.30	3261.47	0.16	0.16	BB	6.1124
33	39.322	48833.11	7829.81	0.38	0.38	BB	6.2368
34	40.014	3851.98	381.78	0.03	0.03	BB	10.0896
35	40.317	4961.12	658.32	0.04	0.04	BB	7.5361
36	42.238	18761.30	2885.47	0.15	0.15	BB	6.5020
37	43.446	13732.95	2227.74	0.11	0.11	BV	6.1645
38	43.677	3641.15	475.12	0.03	0.03	VB	7.6636
39	44.358	10026.73	1381.36	0.08	0.08	BB	7.2586
40	45.172	5679.68	324.72	0.04	0.04	BV	17.4906
41	45.702	2310.12	344.94	0.02	0.02	VV	6.6971
42	46.008	6293.77	986.99	0.05	0.05	VB	6.3768
43	46.372	1949.28	302.87	0.02	0.02	BB	6.4360
44	47.020	2107.15	312.33	0.02	0.02	BV	6.7465
45	47.196	4202.29	663.85	0.03	0.03	VV	6.3302
46	47.619	29472.55	4123.14	0.23	0.23	VB	7.1481
47	48.375	5001.34	702.64	0.04	0.04	BB	7.1179
48	48.899	2159.36	340.40	0.02	0.02	BB	6.3435
49	49.716	18740.77	2850.90	0.15	0.15	BB	6.5736
50	50.618	1643.53	268.59	0.01	0.01	BB	6.1191
51	51.851	4837.78	745.93	0.04	0.04	BB	6.4856
52	52.500	2813.66	340.00	0.02	0.02	BB	8.2754
53	53.374	5142.98	472.31	0.04	0.04	BV	10.8889
54	53.807	5466.45	729.19	0.04	0.04	VB	7.4966
55	54.591	4753.05	633.03	0.04	0.04	BV	7.5084
56	54.847	2941.09	359.05	0.02	0.02	VB	8.1913
57	55.527	5221.12	432.69	0.04	0.04	BV	12.0666
58	55.818	7997.51	987.52	0.06	0.06	VV	8.0966
59	56.119	7917.28	729.16	0.06	0.06	VV	10.8577
60	56.419	9457.81	1323.58	0.07	0.07	VB	7.1456
61	57.425	6079.66	920.87	0.05	0.05	BV	6.6021
62	57.721	3222.87	352.07	0.03	0.03	VB	9.1541
63	58.245	15370.60	2156.61	0.12	0.12	BV	7.1272
64	58.539	3740.16	559.47	0.03	0.03	VB	6.6852
65	59.730	152912.77	20935.39	1.20	1.20	BB	7.3040
66	60.551	5697.23	897.45	0.04	0.04	BB	6.3482
67	61.124	3801.01	592.50	0.03	0.03	BB	6.4152
68	62.465	3837.86	529.91	0.03	0.03	BB	7.2421
69	63.233	3338.14	454.62	0.03	0.03	BV	7.3427
70	63.829	4769.25	503.70	0.04	0.04	VV	9.4684
71	64.103	5798.56	907.53	0.05	0.05	VB	6.3894
72	64.458	11734.34	1579.38	0.09	0.09	BB	7.4297
73	65.313	13346.94	1609.47	0.10	0.10	BB	8.2927
74	66.093	12384.04	1875.33	0.10	0.10	BV	6.6037
75	66.271	8656.41	1211.19	0.07	0.07	VB	7.1470
76	68.129	1588.11	261.75	0.01	0.01	BB	6.0673
77	68.760	9272.45	1062.06	0.07	0.07	BB	8.7306
78	69.233	280420.69	40723.49	2.20	2.20	BB	6.8860
79	69.907	2658.39	387.61	0.02	0.02	BV	6.8585
80	70.166	5251.62	411.17	0.04	0.04	VB	12.7724
81	70.759	525385.06	75061.72	4.12	4.12	BB	6.9994
82	71.769	8112.72	1256.68	0.06	0.06	BB	6.4557
83	74.323	10473.72	1616.43	0.08	0.08	BB	6.4795
84	74.673	23044.18	3610.97	0.18	0.18	BB	6.3817
85	75.404	2704.27	382.70	0.02	0.02	BV	7.0663
86	75.779	30917.48	3929.47	0.24	0.24	VB	7.8681
87	76.994	6822.02	844.73	0.05	0.05	BV	8.0760
88	77.374	5846.20	709.77	0.05	0.05	VB	8.2368
89	79.253	19678.72	2573.63	0.15	0.15	BB	7.6463
90	80.032	29104.16	3690.49	0.23	0.23	BV	7.8863
91	80.349	15186.21	1286.49	0.12	0.12	VV	11.8044
92	80.679	96647.47	14644.64	0.76	0.76	VB	6.5995
93	81.886	3406.81	401.89	0.03	0.03	BV	8.4771
94	82.070	2424.63	404.27	0.02	0.02	VB	5.9976
95	82.567	22425.95	3448.07	0.18	0.18	BV	6.5039
96	82.767	20954.02	2968.91	0.16	0.16	VB	7.0578
97	83.901	8554.66	1032.99	0.07	0.07	BB	8.2815
98	84.435	14576.40	2093.23	0.11	0.11	BV	6.9636
99	84.904	5669.96	616.86	0.04	0.04	VB	9.1916
100	85.370	10592.27	875.19	0.08	0.08	BV	12.1028
101	85.871	5452.31	754.81	0.04	0.04	VB	7.2234
102	87.306	13107.56	1703.26	0.10	0.10	BB	7.6956
103	88.732	18913.37	505.11	0.15	0.15	BB	37.4443
104	89.564	28568.46	3213.56	0.22	0.22	BB	8.8962
105	90.661	53743.43	5959.88	0.42	0.42	BV	9.0175
106	91.069	10654.84	1277.13	0.08	0.08	VB	8.3428
107	91.405	14691.36	1596.74	0.12	0.12	BB	9.2008
108	93.043	7088.27	656.12	0.06	0.06	BB	10.8033
109	95.486	16361.71	1238.22	0.13	0.13	BB	13.2139
110	96.996	6453.01	460.21	0.05	0.05	BB	14.0219
111	99.452	6708.54	542.16	0.05	0.05	BB	12.3737
112	101.918	36381.86	2203.15	0.28	0.28	BB	16.5136
113	103.626	19106.09	981.86	0.15	0.15	BB	19.4590
114	105.248	16733.26	1109.84	0.13	0.13	BB	15.0772
115	106.807	11416.08	768.67	0.09	0.09	BB	14.8518
116	107.401	9238.24	499.96	0.07	0.07	BB	18.4780
		12767494.95	954780.56	100.00	100.00		

Missing Component Report

Component	Expected Retention (Calibration File)

All components were found

Chromatogram

Sample Name : ABS ROSE MAROC   Sample # 157   Page 1 of 2
FileName : E:\TCWS\autoxl\data\
Date : 10/12/2006 1:02:39 PM
Method : laylong   Time of Injection: 10/12/2006 7:12:34 AM
Start Time : 0.00 min   End Time : 122.50 min   Low Point : 4.00 mV   High Point : 54.00 mV
Plot Offset: 4.00 mV   Plot Scale: 50.0 mV

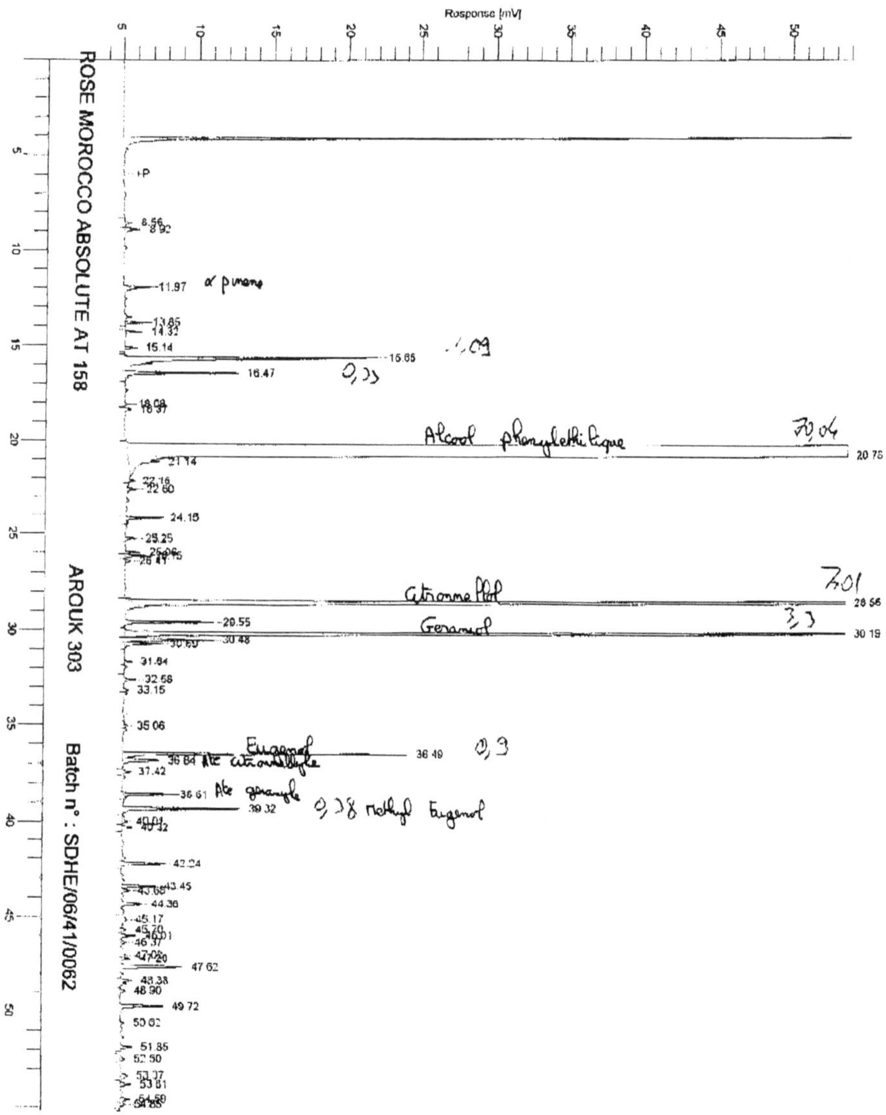

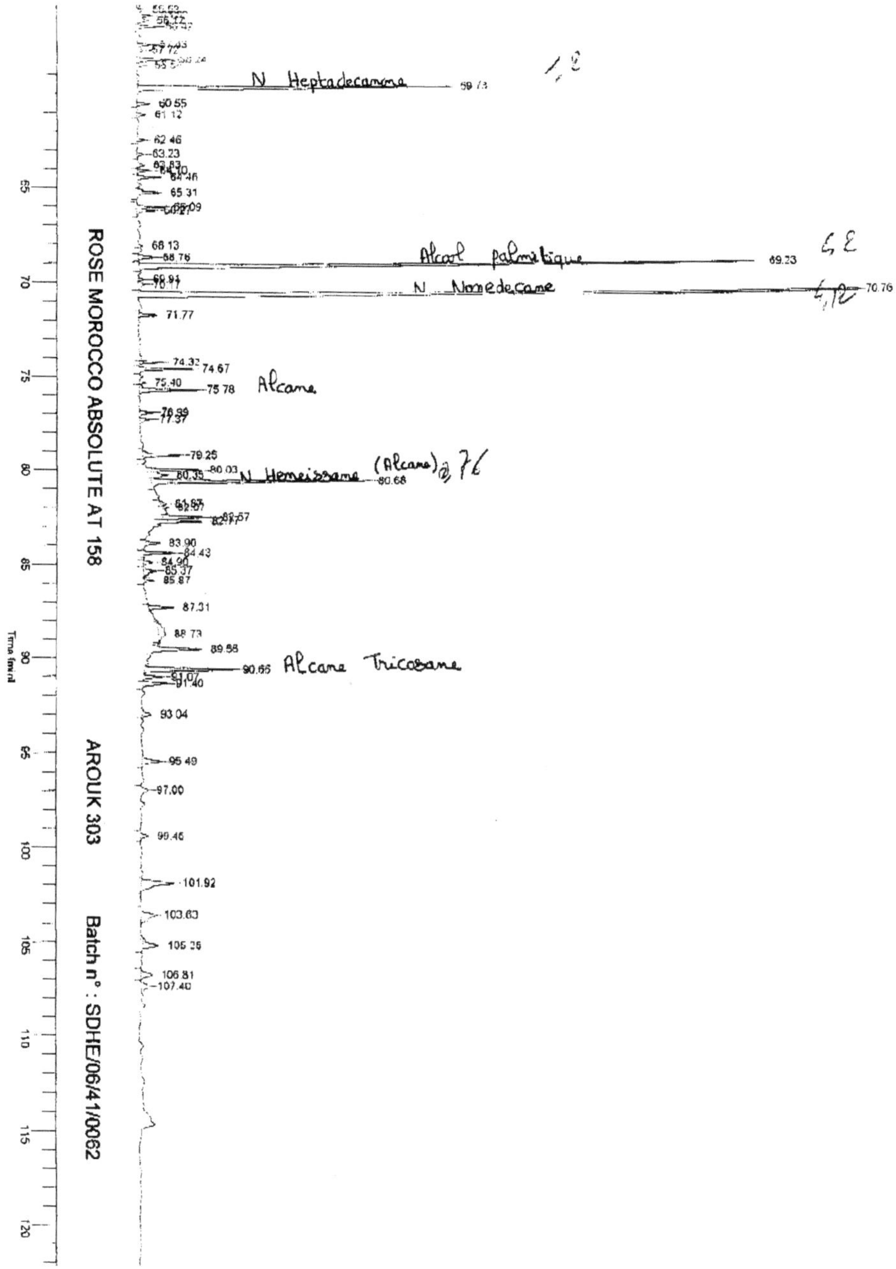
ROSE MOROCCO ABSOLUTE AT 158
AROUK 303
Batch n° : SDHE/06/41/0062
N Heptadecanne
Alcool palmitique
N Nonedecane
Alcane
N Heneissane (Alcane)
Alcane Tricosane

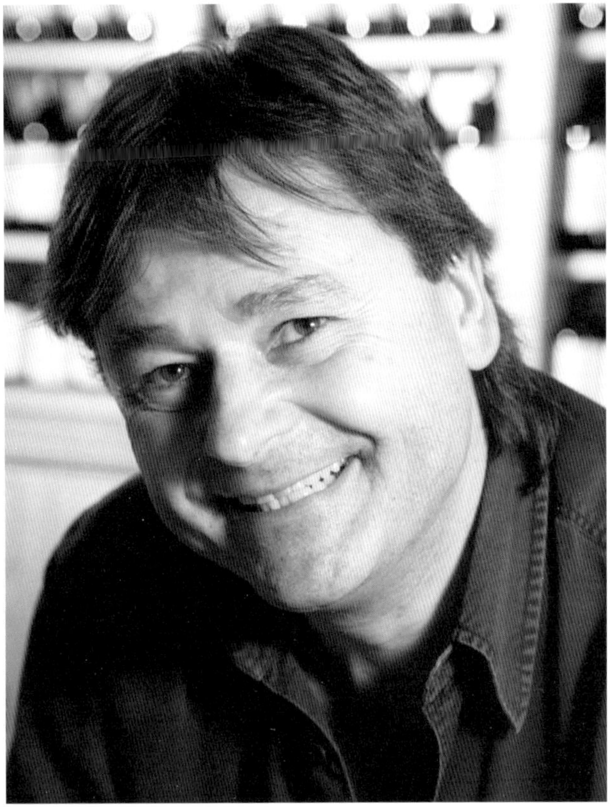

About the Author

Alec Lawless was born in 1958 and grew up round Cheltenham. His father came from Dublin and his mother from a German industrialist family. He had one older brother and two younger sisters one whom later died of motorneuron diesease.

Alec was educated at a number of establishments including Cheltenham Grammar School, Nautical College and HM Prisons Gloucester and Leyhill.

He holds a Dip HE Psychology and a BA in Jungian Psychology, is a trained psychotherapist and has undergone professional wine training.

He loves cooking, music, learning Flamenco guitar, wine, tutoring wine tasting, skiing, motorcycling, reading and studying, travelling and keeping orchids.

At 17 Alec left his family home and went to sea. He was in the merchant navy for three years as a navigation cadet and sailed round the world. After a short stint on cruise ship he jumped ship and went to Reading rock festival.

Back on shore Alec did A-levels at technical college. Then he went to Ireland and did agricultural labouring, followed by a year on oil rigs in the North Sea.

He went to prison for six months for possessing cannabis, spending his 21st birthday inside. Alec says: 'I didn't inhale in case I ever went into politics. Became friends with some interesting people – nuff said.'

On leaving prison he went back to the oil rigs for two years. Then followed a year's unpaid voluntary work, during which he lived in a friend's cellar and helped other friends set up a restaurant in return for food. For the next six years he threw himself into the study of spiritual psychology, visiting monasteries and taking retreats with various Buddhist groups – mostly Zen and Tibetan – plus Jewish mystics, Christians and Sufis. Alec later undertook four years of psychotherapeutic training and has continued doing intensive meditation retreats. He has a deep interest in the relationship between Buddhist models of mind and modern psychology.

He set up a rural community transport scheme covering 52 parishes in the North Cotswolds and was recruited by Wandsworth Community Transport and moved to London. He began Jungian analysis, which lasted for eight years.

Alec left the transport job aged 24 to become full-time student at NE London Polytechnic school of independent study, writing the syllabus for his degree and working as a motorcycle courier for three months.

At weekends and holidays he did relief social work with disturbed and abused children needing psychiatric care. He then took a full-time job with the borough of Hillingdon at a care home for children.

He married in 1987 and left London for rural Gloucestershire. His daughter was born in 1988 and he developed Aqua Oleum a company that specialises in natural aromatic products, which took off and still continues this day.

During this time Alec travelled extensively for cultural reasons – to Tibet, Sikkim, India several times, Nepal, Turkey (Byzantine study trip), Egypt, Palestine, Israel, China and the US.

After twelve years of marriage Alec got divorced and moved to Bristol.

He taught a one-year wine course in Bristol and still does tutored tastings when invited.

In recent years he moved back to rural Gloucestershire, where he now lives with his long-term partner.

Contact Information

For fine fragrances created by Alec, samples and complete supplies for the artisan natural perfumer visit: www.essentially-me.co.uk

You can also visit the showroom where Alec is sometimes available to talk all things smelly. Please email if you have a particular date when you are in Gloucestershire. info@essentially-me.co.uk

Show room address:

Unit 16, Griffin Mill,
London Road,
Thrupp,
Stroud,
Glos
GL5 2AZ.

For pure essential oils, absolutes and aromatherapy supplies please visit: www.aqua-oleum.co.uk

Overseas Distributors

Canada: www.naturatrading.ca
Finland: www.aduki.fi
Norway: www.solaray.no
Japan: www.rimedio-london.com
Korea: www.aqua-oleum.co.kr

Alec is currently working on a range of alcohol free fragrances made in the tradition of attars.

Fragrances created by Alec for Essentially Me

Amber

Heart: masculine floral, Nuance:-balsamic incense, Intrigue :-herbs and spice.

The first impression is soft, warm and masculine. Subtle hints of spice, mint, caraway and thyme evolve on the skin to reveal a floral heart of jasmine, lavender, rose and clary sage. The base is provided by labdanum, frankincense, sandalwood and myrrh with hints of vanilla and patchouli. Distinctive, subtle and masculine.

Chypre

Heart: linden blossom, wood and tobacco, Nuance: floral citrus, Intrigue: marine and hay.

One of the green classics named after Cyprus. A fresh, complex blend of citrus, floral and green notes, which obscure the woody floral heart over the base of tobacco and oak moss. Top citrus notes of linden blossom, neroli, bergamot, lime and cassis gently obscure hints of lavender and rose. Fresh green notes are provided by violet leaf, mint, cumin and seaweed. Cedarwood and cypress help marry the lighter citrus and floral notes with oak moss and tobacco. Like the best men dead butch but also soft and feminine.

Classique

Heart: floral rose, Nuance: citrus, Intrigue: fresh herb and spice.

A classical floral fragrance from yesteryear that whispers elegance. From an era when quality was more important than price. This is timeless, elegant and beautiful. The floral heart is a generous blend of rose Otto, and rose de Mai, supported by orange blossom, neroli and hints of ylang, geranium Bourbon and jasmine. Bergamot, green mandarin and petitgrain provide a subtle citrus lift. Intrigue is imparted by the freshness of coriander and bay, which is warmed by hints of, clove bud and vetivert Bourbon. I had a card from a lady that wears this perfume it said 'this must be very good because all the young men are after me'.

La Joupe

Heart: heady floral, Nuance: Oriental, Intrigue: musky

This is unashamedly musky mysterious and very sexy for the confident woman. Why wait for the young men to chase you? Voluptuous, heady floral notes of tuberose and orange blossoms emerge out of the sultry heart of jasmine, patchouli and ylang. The base is very warm balsamic and musky comprising of vetivert bourbon, frankincense, guaiacwood, labdanum, tonka, oakmoss and vanilla.

White Blooms
Heart: delicate white floral, Nuance: soft green balsam, Intrigue: warm and woody.

A light delicate feminine floral perfume based on mostly white flowers. White champac and orange blossoms cover a faint hint of pink lotus and jasmine. Delicacy is maintained by using absolutes of hay and beeswax to impart soft warm green notes, which are, in turn supported by a base of sandalwood, frankincense and a light vanilla courtesy of benzoin resin. A daytime fragrance delicate enough for warm balmy evenings.

Trade Wind
Heart: cool sea, Nuance: warm earth, Intrigue: warm wind.

A light green day perfume with a citric twist. I wanted to catch the experience of being on an exotic Island. Seaweed absolute with mint and violet leaf conjure up the ocean whilst galbanum resin, sandalwood, and vetivert hint at the soft warm earth. Carried in the breeze are faint impressions of orange flowers, linden blossoms, hay and nutmeg.

Fauve
Heart: vanilla, jasmine, Nuance: rose, sandalwood, Intrigue: patchouli, oakmoss.

Genuine vanilla has tremendous depth and is very sensual. Here we try and show the depth and sensuality which is continents away from the synthetic flavouring. The exotic side is supported by absolutes of jasmine and ylang whilst rose Otto and rose de Mai marry the floral heart to sandalwood and earthy vetivert Bourbon. Mystery comes from oakmoss and patchouli which is softened by frankincense, beeswax abs and trusty absolute of lavender.

Souk
Heart: precious woods, Nuance: rose and spice, Intrigue: incense

This was inspired by travelling in the Middle East and India where there is much to celebrate from these ancient cultures. The haunting smells of the spice markets, the Arab love affair with the rose, fragrant gardens, precious woods, resins and incense. Sandalwood, frankincense and cedar of Lebanon are blended with balsams to provide a complex woody heart. Rose Maroc, jasmine, orris and neroli bring floral tributes from surrounding lands. Citrus fruits, herbs and oriental spices bring nuance from the market stalls and the ancient mysterious opoponax suggests incense with help from frankincense and sandalwood.

Tangos

Heart: violet leaf, tobacco, Nuance: jasmine, rose, Intrigue: guaiacwood.

A bold musky perfume originally made for a friend from Argentina based upon her choices of aromatics (named after the most popular form of Flamenco). It has turned many heads in Buenos Aries. A deep green sultry forest of oak moss, violet leaf, vetivert Bourbon and tobacco slowly releases complex floral bursts from jasmine, ylang, rose Otto, geranium Bourbon, vanilla and rose Maroc with hints of herb, spice hay, coriander and tonka bean.

Kuan Yin

Heart: Osmanthus floral, ***Nuance***: other florals, green notes, citrus, ***Intrigue***: spices and herbs.

Sophisticated, subtle and unusual floral fragrance. Light enough for daytime use and sexy enough for the evening. Named after the Chinese Bodhisattva of compassion whose shrines are often surrounded by pink lotus blossoms. The floral heart is made up of osmanthus with mimosa and is supported by hints of jasmine, pink lotus, white champac, rose and ylang. Nuance and depth are added by using violet leaf and citrus fruit. Finally intrigue is provided by fresh green herbs and spicy tobacco leaf.

Bibliography

Aftel, M. (2001). *Essence and Alchemy.* London: Bloomsbury.

Aravind, A. (2008). *The White Tiger.* London: Atlantic Books.

Curtis, T. & Williams, D (1994). *Introduction to Perfumery.* London: Ellis Horwood.

Groom, N. (1997). *The Perfume Handbook.* London: Blackie Academic and Profesional.

Halliday, J. & Johnson, H. (1992). *The Art and Science of Wine.* London: Mitchell Beazley.

Lawless, J. (1992). *The Encyclopaedia of Essential Oils.* London: Element.

Lefkowith, C. (1994). *The Art of Perfume.* London: Thames and Hudson.

M.Thomas. (2008, May). On Vines and Minds. *The Psychologist* .

Morris, E. (1984). *Fragrance: The Story of Perfume from Cleopatra to Channel.* New York: ET Morris & Co.

Newman, C. (1998). *Perfume, The Art and Science of Scent.* Washington: National Geographic Society.

Sanchez,T. & Turin, L (2008). *Perfumes The Guide.* New York: Viking.

Turin, L. (2006). *The Secret of Scent.* London: faberand faber.

Van Dusen, C. (2007). The Essence of Absence. *Tricycle* , 51--55 & 111-113.

Wiliams, D. (2004). *Perfumes of Yesterday.* New York: Micelle Press.

Index

Page numbers in italics refer to images.